If I Kiss You, Will I Get Diabetes?

BY

Quinn Nystrom

RIVER
PLACE
PRESS

If I Kiss You, Will I Get Diabetes?

BY

Quinn Nystrom

201 West Laurel Street
Brainerd, Minnesota 56401
218.851.4843
www.RiverplacePress.com

Publicity and Representation:
Blue Cottage Agency
www.bluecottageagency.com

First Edition
ISBN Number: 978-0-9831785-8-3
Published and Printed in USA

DEDICATION

To my diabetes heroes who inspired me
to write these pages…

Marcia Meier
Will Nystrom
Emily Wyman Stunek
Ashley Zygmunt

ACKNOWLEDGEMENTS

This book couldn't have happened without the support and help of others.

First, I'm grateful for the American Diabetes Association for giving me the opportunity at the age of sixteen to be their National Youth Advocate for a year. It was through my travels and meeting thousands of incredible people that first inspired the thought for me to do this project. Your faces and your stories are always with me.

I was blessed to work with an incredible team of editors who helped make this book possible; Thor Nystrom, Mark Lindquist, Rachel Reabe Nystrom, and Angela F. Foster. You turned a dream into a reality.

To Krista Rolfzen Soukup of Blue Cottage Agency, Chip and Jean Borkenhagen of River Place Press, thank you for taking a chance on me. You believed in my mission and allowed me to tell my story in a way that was true to me.

To Curt Oltmans and Lisa Falconer, you took a chance encounter and believed a waitress with big dreams could make a difference. I am eternally grateful for your support.

To Honah Kim, you inspired me to be the woman that God has created me to be. You helped me take down the walls to reveal my true, authentic self. This project is a testament to your support, faith, and guidance.

To my dear family, a simple thank you will never be enough for everything that you've done for me. You have been by my side through the journey. I love you Grandma Ruth, Nana, Papa, Mom, Dad, Thor, Will, Roxane, Robin, Becca, Tom, Buck, Linda, Katelyn, Shannon, Eric, and Spencer. You've anchored and encouraged me. Through it all, you loved me, showing me how to love others.

Lastly, I would not be the person I am today without my faith in Jesus Christ. I am blessed to be His and grateful to be walking the path He's set out for me.

Proverbs 3:5-6

FOREWORD

When I was thirteen years old my pancreas shut down forever. At that moment, I became a diabetic. A walking, talking disease condition. I was devastated and desperate. How was I going to get through seventh grade? How was I going to get through the rest of my life?

In my small northern Minnesota town, I didn't know any other teenage girls with diabetes. I was alone and scared to death. A team of health professionals described a complicated regime of four insulin shots a day and provided the latest facts and figures about diabetes. My sympathetic family surrounded me with love and support. But it wasn't enough.

I wanted answers from someone like me who was living with diabetes. Which friends should I tell? When would it get better? Could life be normal with diabetes? There were plenty of books about diabetes, but they didn't answer the questions I was asking. I needed a book that could give it to me straight, that didn't pull any punches. I wanted the truth.

This is the book that I wished I had when I was thirteen years old. It's a story of figuring out how to live with a chronic disease. Over the past decade, I've had the privilege of speaking to audiences across the country. It's a joy to bring a message of hope to others living with diabetes. The big surprise is the number of people without diabetes who tell me the message helped them with their challenges.

I'm hoping this book will provide courage and faith for your journey as it has my own.

Quinn

"Quinn sprang to the national stage at a time when young diabetes advocates were desperately needed. By being herself and channeling her pain into passion, she made a difference in health policy. Her book inspires advocates to strive for greatness and refuse to accept NO for an answer. Failure and challenge, as Quinn shows, can make us better and stronger.

- Dr. Nicole Johnson, Miss America 1999

TABLE OF CONTENTS

Chapter 1   You Get the Choice..6

Chapter 2   Lightning Strikes Twice.....................................10

Chapter 3   The New Normal 16

Chapter 4   From In-Crowd to Outcast............................22

Chapter 5   You Want Me to go to Camp Needlepoint?....28

Chapter 6   Doctor and Patient..34

Chapter 7   Walk a Mile in My Shoes................................38

Chapter 8   Stumbling Blocks to Stepping Stones...........42

Chapter 9   Dateline Diabetes Camps 50

Chapter 10   If I Kiss You Will I Get Diabetes? 56

Chapter 11   Don't Forget the Insulin 60

Chapter 12   Purpose and Passion......................................66

Chapter 13   Ignorance Isn't Bliss 70

Chapter 14   Perfectionists Need Not Apply 74

Chapter 15   Not All Heroes Wear Capes 78

Chapter 16   The Diabetic Food Police 84

Chapter 17   Celebrate the Miles..88

Chapter 18   Diabetes Dating 94

Chapter 19   Dear Quinn..98

Quinn's Mom... 102

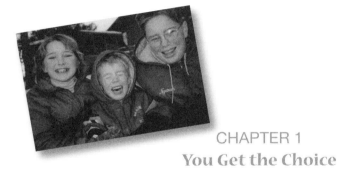

CHAPTER 1
You Get the Choice

I remember the smell of eggs and bacon. The aroma of Dad's coffee drifting into the living room. My parents sat my older brother, Thor, and me down in the formal living room on the stiff, navy couches. It was going to be a serious talk. They never called us in here to deliver good news.

My mom leaned forward and held my hand.

"Your younger brother has diabetes," she said.

She studied my face for a reaction, but I didn't have one. It was like she had told me that a palm tree was growing in the basement. How do you react to something like that?

"Life is going to look a lot different around here now," she continued to say.

Will was five years old. He raced toy cars on the carpet, watched Thomas the Tank Engine, and climbed trees. An incurable illness? My baby brother?

All I knew about diabetes was from the character Stacy in the Baby-sitter's Club book series. When Stacy was out with her friends she would sometimes get shaky and woozy, and they would have to find her a sugary snack to make her feel better.

Will was in preschool. Too young to understand the crushing burden that had just dropped on him. But it's all I thought about. How would his life change? Could he still play in the woods? Would he need to be monitored constantly? Could he still eat the Reese's Puffs cereal that he ran to the kitchen counter for every morning? I also thought, selfishly, could

I still eat the Reese's Puffs in the morning?

There is no easing into diabetes. It's like an unwelcome, demanding visitor barges into the house and refuses to leave. In fact, he makes it clear he will be here every hour and every day for the rest of your life. No wonder they called the disease *die*-abetes. That's exactly what it feels like.

To live, Will has to have insulin shots multiple times a day. A month before Will was diagnosed, I was in for a vaccination. When the doctor came into the room with the shot, I got so dizzy I had to lie down on the cot. Now hypodermic needles will share the kitchen counter with the toaster and bowl of fruit. The insulin vials now take up where the butter shelf was in the refrigerator. The disease state has its own section in our house.

When Dad injected Will's insulin, my father looked far more pained than Will. Dad was calm, but sad, resigned to the life sentence his youngest son had been given.

Will, on the other hand, was the only one in the family who didn't seem destroyed by the diabetes diagnosis. He was the adventurer in our family. The pioneer. Always wanted to try new things. My biggest concern was that his spark—his spontaneity, his energy—would dissolve into an everyday pattern of blood sugar tests and insulin shots. Maybe Will could adjust, but I didn't think I would. Will was the spark plug of the Nystrom house. Without his exuberance, our family would turn into four caretakers and a patient. None of us would be the same. God hadn't been fair to Will. And he hadn't been fair to us. My parents didn't deserve this and neither did Thor and I.

Mourning requires time. We all dealt with the news in different ways, though I'll never know how my parents processed it. They hugged and kissed Will every day and bought all the newest diabetic technology to make his life easier. Once I'd resigned myself to this new life—and stopped feeling sorry for Will and the rest of us—I vowed to make his life easier. I made a promise to myself that I would do everything in my power to make his life as normal as possible.

I got my first chance months later at the Baxter Elementary School's annual fifth grade Inventors' Fair. I wanted to invent a cure for diabetes but had only three weeks to come up with it. Instead, maybe I could make Will's monotonous insulin regime more fun. I had come to hate the boxes of one hundred syringes with their ugly orange tops that were a fixture in the kitchen. Couldn't they come up with a box of multicolored needles? Maybe that could be my invention. Hello, "Hot Shots!" I painted the syringe caps different neon colors. Now, Will had a choice. He still had four shots every single day but he got to choose the colors. At mealtime, Will would look through the box—gold, cobalt, cardinal red, magenta, teal—and choose the one he wanted. It was our little joke. Will, would look at me with his big hazel eyes and toothy grin. "Today is a lime-green day."

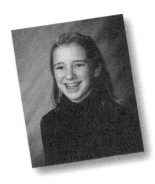

CHAPTER 2
Lightning Strikes Twice

Surviving middle school as a thirteen-year-old is a full-time occupation. The key is conformity. One wrong move, one original thought, one lapse in groupthink, is all it takes to be voted off the island—or eat lunch alone in the cafeteria. Thankfully, everyone wore braces or I would have served a life sentence of an overbite.

Our cross-country ski banquet was held on a cold, windy evening in March. My friends and I sat at long tables with fixed benches and listened to our coaches praise our teamwork. In Minnesota, you figure out what you have to do to survive the endless winters, and cross-country skiing provided lots of time with friends. I was not the fastest or slowest skier, just a content member of the middle of the pack.

The buffet of takeout pizza and sheet cake upset my stomach. I returned to the back of the cafeteria for another cup of punch, but I was still thirsty. During the presentation for outstanding skier of the year, I went into the hallway to find a drinking fountain.

When we arrived home, I poured a large tumbler of water and downed it. When I looked up, my mom was watching me.

"Quinn, would you check your blood sugar on Will's blood glucose meter?"

"Why in the world would I do that?"

"I saw you get up during the banquet a couple of times to get something more to drink. I'm worried. It's probably nothing, but I want to check your blood sugar."

Was she crazy? After Will was diagnosed with diabetes, my mom turned into a diabetes vigilante. The doctor told her our family would be featured on the cover of the *New England Journal of Medicine* if her other children developed type 1 diabetes. After all, we had no family history of diabetes. Like all moms, long odds didn't prevent her from worrying.

Mom stood by the kitchen drawer containing Will's diabetes supplies. It was clear that I would not be leaving the kitchen without a glucose check. She squeezed my finger. A quick prick with the lancet produced a small drop of blood. Thirty seconds seemed like thirty minutes as we watched the glucose machine count down to the results. The house was quiet. Will was in bed. Thor was in his downstairs bedroom, and Dad was watching sports from his favorite spot on the leather couch in the family room. The small display window on the pocket-sized meter finally flashed its result, but instead of a number, it produced a pair of letters. We stood together with our eyes locked on the word "HI."

Without a word, I ran down the stairs to my room. I refused to let my mind consider what HI might mean. After two years and 3 months of helping Will monitor his blood sugar, I knew that a healthy glucose reading was between 80 and 120. When he was first diagnosed, his blood sugar had been 600, the top number the meter could display. Above that, it flashes HI—a possible death sentence.

I was already in my pink plaid flannel pajamas under the covers when my mom and dad knocked on my bedroom door. One look at my father and I knew there was no going back. His big, brown eyes brimmed with love and compassion, just like a big teddy bear.

As a pharmacist, my dad managed Will's diabetic regimen as he did so many of his customers. Dad had already called our pediatrician who directed him to give me a shot of ten units of short-acting insulin and report to the clinic first thing the next morning. As he advanced toward me holding the needle, I could hardly breathe. It was the family joke that Will was the only Nystrom who could handle hypodermic needles. My dad pulled up my sleeve and plunged the needle into my arm, all the while murmuring reassurances. "We'll get to the bottom of this. Don't worry. Everything is going to be okay. You are going to be fine." In short, the same kind of crap they were probably telling the passengers on the Titanic after it hit the iceberg.

I could not wait until they left the room. I grabbed the phone and called my best friend, Stina.

"It's Quinn. Something terrible has happened. It's horrible."

"What is it? Just say it."

"I think I have diabetes, just like Will."

"How do you know that?" Stina said. "We were just at the ski banquet. You looked normal."

I started to cry. Just saying it out loud was hideous.

"My mom just checked my blood sugar and it's sky-high. The meter can't even read the number. Do you think I'm going to die?"

Stina is straightforward and tells it like it is whether you like it or not. It's her best and worst quality. "You are not going to die. No matter what. Stay positive. Whatever happens, I'm still your best friend."

My mind bounced between the best and worst scenarios. It was a mistake. The meter was broken. The meter wasn't broken. I am no longer a thirteen-year-old girl. I am a disease condition. Will seems to have survived three years with diabetes, but he's stronger than I am. He plays hockey, hangs out with friends, and is one of the happiest kids I know. I will be rejected. My life is over.

The next morning, March 17, 1999, we got into the car to go to the doctor's office. The nurse showed us into the small examination room. I was praying that all of this was a terrible mistake. I begged God to perform a miracle. The nurse poked my finger, centered the drop of blood on a small strip, and left the room.

Five minutes later, Dr. Stevens, sporting his trademark bow tie under a lab coat, joined us in the exam room. He stepped forward with a big smile and shook my hand.

"Your blood work shows that you, in fact, have type 1 diabetes. As you know, this is a chronic illness, but you can live a full life by managing your blood sugar with insulin injections."

I didn't look at the doctor. I didn't look at my mom or dad. I looked at my hands and tried to breathe in and out, in and out.

"What questions do you have?" The doctor had his back to my parents, focusing his attention on me. I had no questions. I had no thoughts. I had no future.

My parents were as stunned as I was. My father, a pharmacist, asked about what type of insulin I would be taking, the meter that I would use, and the necessary medical questions.

My mom stared at the doctor in disbelief and asked, "Will Quinn be going straight to the hospital from here?"

Dr. Stevens said it wouldn't be necessary because we were well accustomed to living with diabetes and monitoring blood sugars.

The small room smelled of deep-cleaning agents and the only sound in the room was the paper crunching under me on the exam table as I crossed my legs.

This is not going to change my life. This is not going to change my life, I thought. Will is living a normal life and I will too. I'm normal, I'm normal, I'm normal. Nothing is wrong. I feel fine.

I asked Dr. Stevens through my pink and purple braces the first question that came to my mind, "Can I go to the seventh grade dance tonight at the YMCA?"

After a few awkward moments, the doctor said yes, including the caveat I would hear the rest of my life, "If you manage your blood sugars properly, there is really nothing you can't do."

We walked silently through the snow-covered parking lot to the car. We had been in the clinic for such a short time that the car was still warm. As Dad backed out of the parking spot, my mom suggested I take the day off from school. Her expression was uneasy, unable to gauge my reaction.

That was the last thing I wanted to do. Nothing had changed. I was going straight back to school and then to the dance. I would wear my Silver blue jeans and pink Tommy Hilfiger shirt. I wasn't sick. I wanted to get away from my parents and their anxious eyes.

"Drop me off at the front door," I said. "I'm fine, and I'll see you after school. Don't worry about me." I hung on to the one thread of hope I heard from the doctor. He assured me there would be a cure for diabetes before I left for college. If I could just hang on for five years, everything would be back to normal.

I can do that. Diagnosis is a nightmare, but diabetes has an end date. I will reach it. I will live to see a cure. It's coming.

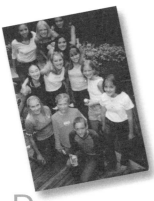

CHAPTER 3
The New Normal

Dad pulled our tan Suburban to the curb in front of Mississippi Horizons Middle School, perched on a hill overlooking the Mississippi River in Brainerd, Minnesota. Most days, the morning drop-off involved dodging buses, bikes, and a steady stream of cars. Today, it was just Dad, Mom, and me. I had already missed two classes, but I was determined to be on time for lunch, the social highlight of every school day.

Although it seems in hindsight slightly melodramatic, two words continued to scroll across my mental screen: Death Sentence. Death Sentence.

I'm going to die. He said I'm going to die. Of course, he hadn't actually said that, I reminded myself. To break up the steady stream of negative thoughts, I changed the monotonous words in my head: Nothing has changed, Quinn. Nothing has changed. Nothing has changed. Nothing has changed.

I looked at my palms. They were the same. I was wearing the same gold necklace my grandmother gave me a few Christmases ago, as I did every day. My pink chipped fingernails were the same. My Lucky jeans were the same.

Nothing has changed, Quinn. Nothing has changed.

All I wanted to do was wave my parents good-bye, assure them I'd be all right, and rush to my usual seat between Allison and Jillian in the cafeteria. It would be, I thought, the first normal thing I had done that day. But no, my parents insisted we meet with the school nurse. My mom was working hard to be casual, trying to keep me calm.

"It won't take long, Quinn. We have to explain what the doctor said, so that they're aware of it. It's no big deal. Parents of kids with asthma do the same thing."

We walked into the school together and went straight to the office. My father told Mrs. Hopper, the school nurse, that we had just come from the clinic where I had been diagnosed with type 1 diabetes. I studied the fabric of my jeans. There was nothing I wanted to see less than pity from Mrs. Hopper. I didn't even want her to know. I didn't want anyone to know. I pretended I was already in the cafeteria with my gang as the three of them discussed how I would check my blood sugar in school.

Nothing has changed. Nothing has changed.

It didn't even seem like they were talking about me. I felt like I had been invited into an intense meeting in which my parents and a nurse were discussing a sister I never knew I had. I felt bad for this mysterious girl. Glucose, needles, insulin—did she even know what was in store for her?

My mother was now insistent, "Are you sure you don't want to just take the day off of school and go home and rest?"

"I'm fine. Don't worry about me."

If anyone saw my parents in the hallways, I would need to give a long explanation about why they were there. I had to get them out of the building immediately.

"I'm fine. See you later." What a relief to see them walk away and be freed from their careful watch.

I rushed to my locker and grabbed my science book. The class was working on a science project when I slipped into the room. Allison looked up and said, "Where were you?" Brittany made a joke that I had overslept so I could get beauty sleep for the dance that night. I told them I was at the doctor's office.

"What for?" Brittany asked.

I stood still. What was I going to tell them? Stupid. Maybe I should just tell them that it was a regular checkup. My friends didn't need to know the truth.

Three years before, when my five-year-old brother was diagnosed with diabetes, we were at Thor's orchestra concert at Tornstrom Auditorium. The audience had settled into their seats and the lights were just dimming when Will yelled, "I have diabetes." He said it in the same tone that an umpire would yell, "Play ball!"

He was so proud of himself. My mother clamped her hand over his mouth and the people around us turned and smiled. That is exactly what I wasn't capable of—owning a label. Will was the kind of kid who wore weird clothes to school for the fun of it. He didn't care what anybody thought. He was cool without trying.

I looked at the beaker on the table next to Brittany and briefly considered diverting her attention and asking what chemicals the class was mixing that day. Instead, perhaps motivated by the idea that I could be as confident as my younger brother, I blurted, "I was diagnosed with type 1 diabetes, just like Will. Please don't tell anyone." I turned away before I could see her face. I opened my textbook, hiding my face. I might as well have stood on my chair in class and yelled out my announcement.

Before class ended, I was called down to the office. Mrs. Hopper met me.

"You will need to stop by every day before lunch so you can check your blood sugar and give yourself a shot. I'll be there to help you," she said.

How embarrassing. I had zero intention of following that rule. Why not just announce at the next all-school assembly that Quinn Nystrom was a freak? Mrs. Hopper demonstrated how to prick my finger to get a drop of blood. Didn't she know I'd been helping Will test his blood sugar for over two years? Four times a day, every day. That was over one thousand times total.

When you have diabetes, there are no vacation days.

That's when it hit me. Just like that, knowing there would be no hiding my disease, knowing I would never again have a day when I could eat my favorite Hot Tamales candy and drink Mountain Dew without checking my blood sugar and taking an insulin shot.

I wasn't alone in Mrs. Hopper's office. Clark was there checking his blood sugar. I remembered seeing him at the annual Walk for Diabetes held every fall in Brainerd. He and his pals wore black T-shirts and a matching attitude. I remembered that he was diagnosed as a toddler. Clark and Will were lucky, I thought. They began their careers in diabetes before they knew what life could be like without it. Unfortunately, I realized what I was going to have to give up.

He was a nice guy, but he was just repeating what everyone was saying, from my parents to the doctors to Mrs. Hopper.

"Everything is going to be okay."

He was a nice guy, but he was just repeating what everyone was saying, from my parents to the doctors to Mrs. Hopper.

Nothing is going to be okay, I wanted to shout.

I grabbed the school lunch of the day: meat casserole, pineapple, skim milk, and a marble cake with green frosting celebrating St. Patty's Day. The lunchroom hummed with talk and laughter. My friends were in deep conversation about that night's school dance when I arrived at the round, blue table with my tray. It was suddenly quiet. Please, don't ask any questions, I thought. Let me just sit down and eat my lunch. Please, don't say anything.

I dropped my tray and Brittany grabbed my piece of cake.

"Who wants Quinn's cake?" she said. "She can't eat sugar anymore because she has diabetes."

My face flamed and I heard a roar in my ears. A couple of the girls giggled nervously, watching my face for a reaction. I focused on the middle crease of the table as tears surfaced. I blinked quickly to keep them from falling. A couple of girls pushed their forks toward my plate to grab a bite of my cake.

Kate, my best friend, saved me. "Guess who Quinn is going to the dance with?"

The awkward moment passed. I mechanically ate. I tried to act like I was interested in what Allison, Brittany and Jill were wearing to the dance.

"Will Chad be there?" I heard myself say.

Somebody answered, I think.

"Where are we going to meet?" I said when they stopped talking.

Just pretend, Quinn.

Act normal. Pretend you are normal.

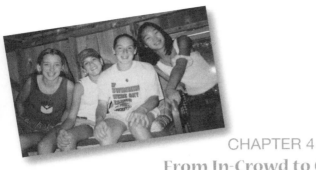

CHAPTER 4
From In-Crowd to Outcast

I survived a week with an incurable disease. Nothing was the same. Seven days down, and eighty years to go. I had to stop thinking about it. Pretend everything was normal. I wish it were that easy. Why did it happen to me? Why did it happen to Will? It was like winning the lottery, against all odds. Only in this case, it was not a lottery, it was a double death sentence for Will and me. Even worse than death, it was a life in prison.

Will didn't seem bothered about diabetes. He was living his eight-year-old life with enthusiasm. What was wrong with him? What was wrong with me? I thought we could at least complain together. But it wasn't happening. Will was born an optimist. His advice, based on three years of diabetes under his belt: "Forget about it. Who cares?"

The only person I knew with diabetes, other than Will, was my great-grandma. She was diagnosed with type 2 diabetes when she was in her eighties. Her pancreas still worked but needed some help. The last time we visited her in Florida, Mom filled her syringes every few days. I sat at the table while my mom stuck each needle into a tiny bottle of insulin. She put the filled needles in a glass decorated with large oranges and stuck them in the refrigerator. I got the creeps every time I saw them sitting next to the milk carton. Luckily, Oma gave herself the shots when I wasn't around.

Oma was ninety-two years old and living in a nursing home. It was sad. The nurses were probably still sticking her with insulin. What a future I had to look forward to. Needles, needles and then, when I'm an old lady, more needles.

I hated math but just had to figure out how many shots I had to look forward to if I lived to ninety-two. I gave myself four shots a day. If I lived to be ninety-two, that meant that I had 115,340 shots ahead of me. I was thirteen years old and my life was over before it had even started.

With great effort, I forced myself back to the present. American History class bored me senseless. Class had just started when my assigned seatmate got up to talk to our teacher, Mr. Johnson. Instead of the usual single chair/desk combo, our history room had small tables with two chairs. It was dumb, because we weren't doing scientific experiences or group projects. We had been in these seats for three months, and Jacob was okay. He wasn't nice, but he wasn't mean either.

Jacob walked back to our desk and sat down without looking at me. After class, Mr. Johnson asked if he could see me. I went up to his desk, wondering if I had bombed last week's test. Mr. Johnson glanced at me and then cleared his throat. "Jacob has asked to change seats," he said, looking down at his hands. "He heard that you have diabetes and is concerned that it could be contagious."

Blood rushed to my head. I looked at Mr. Johnson stone faced, but my mind was roaring. How did Jacob find out? He didn't even know my last name. Only a handful of my closest friends knew that I had been diagnosed with diabetes. Now the whole school knew?

I wanted to die.

I can't do this.

I won't do this.

Jacob is an idiot. Even a fool knows diabetes isn't contagious. Mr. Johnson should have sent Jacob to the principal's office for a verbal beating. Last week I had friends and a life and a future.

When I was capable of speaking, I told Mr. Johnson I hated sitting next to Jacob and would gladly change seats. He indicated I could choose between two empty tables in the back of the room. It was the beginning of my exile—sentenced to solitary confinement because I was stupid enough to get this stupid disease. The doctor told me repeatedly that I didn't cause it. I couldn't prevent it. It just happened. That makes me the unluckiest person on the planet. Welcome to my new life.

My friends did everything they could to help me get through my nightmare. Most of them were longtime friends from elementary school. We'd grown up together. At lunch I asked them if everyone in the school knew I had diabetes. "Well," Ashlee said. "Probably not everybody." The others looked down at their trays.

"Just screw them," Laura replied. "Who cares what they think anyway?"

Easy for her to say.

I remember having a terrible fight with my best friends in third grade. They ganged up on me about some dumb thing. When I got off the bus, my mom was sitting on our log-swing on the lawn waiting for me. She asked me how school was and I said fine, not cracking a smile. I crawled up on the top of the swing and stretched out along the log. Mom was yapping on about something when she felt a drop of rain. She looked up and realized it was my tears dropping right on her head. That's how I felt that day in history class. I was on my own. I couldn't count on any-one. They didn't understand and they would never understand.

I felt lonely even when I was with my best friends. Instead of being grateful for them, I focused on the Jacobs of the world. Some were mean and some were just dumb. I think I knew that the majority of people were kind, but diabetes was the beginning of a lonely stretch in my life.

A month went by and life did not return to normal, but it sort of looked like normal from the outside. I had joined the golf team at school with a handful of friends, and we were looking forward to missing school for out-of-town meets. Lauren's birthday was coming up, and she was celebrating with a slumber party. It was going to be really fun. The party would be at a big resort on Gull Lake that her grandparents owned.

When I told my parents, they exchanged a quick glance and said we would have to figure out how it would work. Are you kidding? What was there to work out?

My dad said to me calmly, "You can go, but you have to call before meals and snacks with your blood sugar numbers so I can calculate the insulin doses."

It wouldn't be a big deal, they said. I could just make a phone call to Mom before supper and then sneak away to the bathroom with my needle and insulin.

It seemed miserable, but it would be a night away from my parents' watchful eyes. Freedom! (My brothers' favorite cry after watching *Braveheart* multiple times.) Mom told me she had called Lauren's mom and there would be special snacks and treats that were "diabetic-friendly." No more regular Mountain Dew for me. How awkward. I was beyond mortified. I thought about just staying home but knew it would look worse to not go.

All week at lunch, we talked about the upcoming slumber party. These gatherings were the highlights of our social life. Friday, I packed my sleeping bag and my diabetic essentials, and my mom drove me to the resort on Gull Lake. She reminded me of our agreed upon phone schedule and wished me a fun and safe night. Her voice was cheerful, but her eyes looked kind of worried. I didn't care. I was on my own.

Once inside, the twelve of us set up camp, unrolling sleeping bags and placing our pillows. It was so much fun to be at the resort and have a big room for the party. I unrolled my purple flannel sleeping bag with the plaid lining next to Jillian. She was my tennis partner and one of my best friends. She looked worried.

"Quinn, you can't sleep by me!"

"Why not?" I said.

"Because I don't want to wake up next to a dead person."

"What in the world are you talking about?"

"My mom told me that people with diabetes can go into comas while they sleep at night. That freaks me out. I don't think I would even be able to sleep because I would be looking at you all night."

I tried to laugh. "You're nuts." But in my mind I just kept repeating,

I'm the same person, I'm the same person, I'm the same person. I would never treat my friends this way no matter what disease they had. How would she feel if she were the one with diabetes? I couldn't even fit in with my best friends. I think it would be easier to move to a new town with a new school with new people who had no idea I had diabetes.

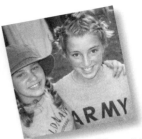

CHAPTER 5
You Want Me to go to Camp Needlepoint?

Being thirteen years old is hideous for almost everyone. Being thirteen and diagnosed with an incurable and chronic illness is almost unbearable. The only way I knew how to cope with diabetes was to ignore it as much as possible. I didn't want to talk about it or think about it. My goal was to keep it locked up in a very small box. My friends got the picture and didn't bring the subject up. I sneaked off to check my blood sugar and give myself an insulin shot and then returned to my real life. My parents would ask me how I was doing, feeling, coping.

"Just fine, no problem," I would say.

Discussion closed. If I let my feelings escape the box, I was afraid I would have a breakdown.

A few months after my diagnosis, my mom brought up the subject of summer camp. I perked up. I loved going to camp—packing up your stuff, moving into a rustic cabin, making new friends and, most of all, being on your own without parents telling you what to do. I had been to Camp Shamineau every summer since second grade. Stretching along the shore of a beautiful lake about an hour from home, Shamineau had it all—horses, bonfires, crafts, and lots of new people to meet.

Mom talked about a new camp she read about in Wisconsin that offered sailing and rock climbing. It sounded great until she mentioned it was a diabetes camp. "I think it would be a great opportunity for you to meet other kids with diabetes," she explained. "Camp Needlepoint sounds perfect."

Did she really say Camp *Needlepoint?* Is this some kind of sick joke? Throwing a bunch of kids with diabetes together at a place called Needlepoint? No thanks. That is the last place on earth I would go. I would rather work on a prison chain gang cleaning ditches for the summer. Unfortunately, that was not an option.

"It's bad enough to have diabetes, but now you are going to ruin my summer by forcing me to a camp for diabetics?" I slammed down my beach bag on the counter.

"I don't want to sit around and learn about needles and complications and why my dumb pancreas broke down. I don't care. I hate this. I hate my life."

I sneaked a quick look at my mom to see if she was wavering. Her eyes were full of sympathy, but her mouth was set in a straight line. Mom often told us that her job was not to be our friend but our mother. I could tell diabetes camp was in my future, ready or not.

"You're going to Camp Needlepoint this summer. It's only seven days and I think it will be good for you." Mom had that look on her face. The one that said, subject closed. My summer ruined.

Camp Needlepoint was going to end out my summer. I tried to forget about it and hang out with my friends. We played tennis, rode our bikes, listened to *N SYNC and the Backstreet Boys' newest summer hits, and sunbathed on the dock. There was a lot of discussion about boys and what eighth grade would be like. I didn't tell anyone about the dreaded Needlepoint. How embarrassing. My friends thought I was leaving for a family vacation in late August.

Packing for Needlepoint was just like packing for Shamineau—sleeping bag and pillow, shorts, swimsuit, sweatshirt, and tennis shoes. I imagined a nurse in a white uniform passing out the medical textbooks and the syringes after we got there.

My mom must have been afraid I would jump out of the car on the drive to Needlepoint, so she brought her sister along for reinforcement. Aunt Roxane has always been one of my favorite grown-ups. A year younger than my mom, she was at the hospital the day I was born. We were tight. When the parents went haywire, I turned to Roxane for sympathy and support. She was a great listener and willing to negotiate with my mom on my behalf. Roxane was almost always on my side, but she agreed with Mom. She thought meeting other kids my age with diabetes would be a good thing.

It was a long, four-hour ride to Hudson, Wisconsin. My mom and aunt chatted most of the way. I sat in silence in the backseat. The last thing I wanted was to be identified as a diabetic. Now I was being forced to go somewhere with 200 kids that all had diabetes. I couldn't bear the thought of having to sit around a campfire and talk about having this chronic disease. I made my mom promise she would pick me up at the earliest possible time on the last day of camp. I was already counting down the hours.

We arrived just before lunch on Saturday. The camp stretched along a bluff overlooking the St. Croix River. Kids were lined up getting their cabin assignments. It really didn't look that different than Camp Shamineau. Not a needle in sight. When we got to the front of the line, a college guy pointed out the platform tents on the map where the teenagers stay. "You guys are going to have a blast," he said. He must have noticed how nervous I was.

"Where do we have the lectures?" I asked.

He just laughed. "Sorry to disappoint you. No lectures. Just a lot of fun."

I said good-bye to my mom and aunt and slowly walked toward a pair of purple platform tents on the edge of the woods. Inside the empty girls' tent, I unrolled my sleeping bag on a top bunk. I couldn't hold back the tears. This was not the life I had imagined. I didn't know how I was going to survive the seven days.

A girl, around my age, walked into the tent and crawled up on my bed.

"Hi, my name is Nicole. I'm from Babbitt, Minnesota. Where are you from?"

I choked back the tears and said, "The Brainerd Lakes area."

"Cool. I come to camp every year and just love it. We're going to be the best of friends."

She jumped down and went to set up her bunk next to mine. Nicole seemed so normal. She was pretty, with blond curls, big, blue eyes, and dimples—the girl at school that all the guys would want to date. What was she doing here? But wait. She had diabetes, just like me? She seemed so happy and carefree. Nicole didn't say anything about diabetes. She was talking nonstop about the fun we were going to have.

"This is my favorite week of the year," Nicole said. "Finally, we are old enough to be in tents with guys right next door!"

Another girl walked in eating Starbursts. She was popping them into her mouth, one after another. She said her name was Breanna. I looked again, and yes, she was eating candy. I remembered the day I was diagnosed, when a friend at school announced that I would never be able to eat sugar.

"Aren't you going to get in trouble for bringing candy?" I asked her.

Breanna looked up at me and said, "Just because you have diabetes doesn't mean you can't ever eat candy."

During the seven days of camp, we had a blast learning about rock climbing and sailing. We played jokes on each other and stayed up late talking. Nicole and I decided we were twins separated at birth. We even slept together in the same bunk bed so we could talk about our "diacrushes" (the guys at camp we were crushing on that day). Nicole and I made plans to return the following summer and sign up for the sailing camp that included a trip on Lake Superior. We figured out how far Babbitt was from Baxter and when we could get together.

My mom arrived at Needlepoint at 10:00 a.m. the following Saturday as promised. She was shocked when I told her I didn't want to leave and couldn't wait to come back next summer. She and Nicole's mother had to practically pull us apart. That week, Nicole taught me that I could still be me, even if I did have diabetes.

The weird thing about diabetes camp was that diabetes was not the focus. The disease that had loomed so large in my life since the day I was diagnosed, was really no big deal at Needlepoint. When I saw the young campers running and laughing and playing, I was ashamed of myself. They figured it out a lot sooner than I had. When I stopped long enough to think about it, the four shots of insulin I gave myself every day took a total of ten minutes at the most. That leaves twenty-three hours and fifty minutes that are available for living.

I had wasted so much time being ashamed of something I had no control over. My pancreas just quit. So what? Get over it and get on with it. I would not feel sorry for myself anymore. Life was out there and it was time to get back to it.

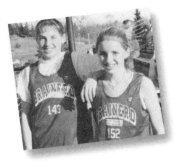

CHAPTER 6
Doctor and Patient

My Minnesota hometown is a dead ringer for Garrison Keillor's mythical Lake Wobegon. The Mississippi River flows through the middle of town and it's almost true: "All the women are strong, all the men are good-looking and all the children are above average." My dad and his dad and his dad's dad are all from here. The Swedish immigrants thought it looked like home. Brainerd is a great name for a town. Our debate team uses the slogan "We put the *Brain* in Brainerd." The Knowledge Bowl team prefers, "We put the *Nerd* in Brainerd."

Living in Brainerd had its advantages, but it didn't offer the medical options we needed. With two children with type 1 diabetes, my parents were looking for a diabetes specialist to work with our pediatrician. Their search for an endocrinologist, a medical doctor who specializes in the diagnosis and treatment of diabetes, led them to the International Diabetes Center in Minneapolis, just two and a half hours south of us. I didn't care. I hated thinking about diabetes, talking about diabetes, or even acknowledging having diabetes. What was the point of driving half a day to see a doctor? The only positive thing was a day off of school and my parents' promise that I could choose where we would have lunch.

But I was wrong. It made a huge difference to see doctors who specialized in treating young people with diabetes. They understood. On my first visit to the IDC, I met an angel, Diabetes Nurse Educator Marcia Meier. She had a head full of dark curls, mod glasses, and a lab coat covering a bright pink sweater. Her desk was crowded with toys, gizmos, and doodads she allowed me to play with while we talked. This was not the usual "doctor talks, patient listens" scene. She asked me how I was doing and then she listened. Marcia was honest about the challenges of living with diabetes. Even at the young age of thirteen, she made me feel as if I could do it. Yes, there was a lot to learn and a lot to think about, but she promised things would get easier. My life would go on.

Nothing has changed, I thought. For the first time, I actually believed it.

I felt comfortable asking Marcia questions that were important to me.

"My parents are nervous about me sleeping over at a friend's house," I said. "How can I persuade them to let me go? Does everyone have to know I have diabetes?"

"Just because you have diabetes doesn't mean your life is over," Marcia counseled. "Don't think too far ahead. Take one day, one task, at a time."

As the years passed, I often called Marcia on pressing matters.

"How and when should I tell my college roommate that I have diabetes and will have to store insulin in our refrigerator?"

"I'm wearing a close-fitting, green silk dress to Christmas Ball. Where can I put my insulin pump?" After much debate about fabric and undergarments we came up with a solution.

"I've heard from other patients that wearing Spanx under a dress is a great way to hold and hide the pump," responded Marcia.

In my late twenties, I found myself living in Minneapolis, trying to adjust to a full-time job and an independent life. I traveled five thousand miles per month as a salesperson, working for a pharmaceutical distributor helping manage specialty pharmacies.

I made an appointment with Marcia and she suggested I try a diabetes support group. "Are you kidding?" I said. "People my age don't do support groups." My life was humming along. Job. Check. House. Check. Good control of my diabetes. Check. I could imagine a roomful of weeping, desperate types hugging each other. No thanks.

Marcia urged me to give it a try. As always, she was right.

It was a group of men and women with type 1 diabetes, from eighteen to fifty years old. It brought me back to the happy days at Camp Needlepoint where we could talk freely about the challenges of diabetes. We could get honest feedback from our peers. What do you guys think about the latest insulin pump to hit the market? When do you tell a guy you are diabetic? Does your employer have to know?

Diabetes can be a lonely experience. The public has misconceptions about diabetes, and sometimes I think it's easier to play "good diabetic." I remember being out for business dinners and just getting chicken and vegetables and passing on the starches because I didn't want any "food police" comments on my food selection. The group helped me understand I wasn't helping anybody by doing this. My fellow diabetics helped me become more comfortable with living with diabetes. And, as they put it, "grow thicker skin" when it came to an outsider's ignorant comments. We had a lot of good laughs about "helpful advice" from acquaintances with a working pancreas.

In college, I went to three different endocrinologists before I found one who was a good fit. I had to find somebody I could be honest with and have the freedom to share what was working and what wasn't. I'm shocked at people who stay with their doctor, not because the relationship is working, but because it would be too awkward to switch.

I've been with my current endocrinologist for seven years. We have an open and honest relationship. It didn't start that way. I needed to feel comfortable that she wouldn't criticize me if I messed up. It's important to have an open dialogue with your doctor, but it's also a process. Over several appointments, I realized I could trust her. She praised me when things were going well and encouraged me to work harder when they weren't. An iron fist was not going to motivate me. When she was away on maternity leave and returned, I asked her how her insulin pump worked during her pregnancy.

"I don't have diabetes!" she answered.

We both had a good laugh. She had been so kind and compassionate to me over the years, I assumed she too was a type 1 diabetic.

Diabetes is a dynamic disease and it's important to keep up to date on the latest research and treatment options. Find a doctor who wants you to be part of the team. If the doctor prefers to lecture instead of listen, keep looking. Ask around and find out whom others recommend. You can check the Internet. Reach out on social media sites for endocrinologists and diabetes nurse-educators who specialize in treating young people with diabetes. Audition your doctor. See if the relationship is going to work and then feel free to move on if it doesn't. If you won't stand up for yourself, you'll never receive the care and compassion you deserve.

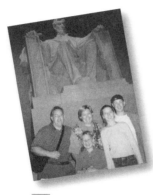

CHAPTER 7
Walk a Mile in My Shoes

The first summer I had diabetes, my parents and I attended a workshop for parents of teenagers with diabetes at the International Diabetes Center in St. Louis Park, Minnesota. I was not thrilled when we filed into an auditorium to listen to experts blab on about "the disease." I tuned out. Frankly, I knew everything I needed to know about diabetes. The disease sucks. I have it. And that's the end of the story.

It was day two of the five-day seminar when my ears perked up. The speaker was addressing himself to the teenagers in the room.

"Do you think your parents really know how tough it is to manage diabetes?" he asked. "How do you think they would handle this disease?"

A ripple of laughter spread across the auditorium.

"Poof, now both of your parents have been diagnosed with type 1 diabetes," the speaker proclaimed. "For the next twenty-four hours they will monitor their blood sugar and give themselves shots."

Parents all over the room were shaking their heads and whispering. A nurse entered the room with a cart filled with blood sugar kits, test strips, lancets, syringes, bottles of saline solution (to stand in for insulin), and logbooks.

"The parents will now be the patients," the nurse explained, looking out over the small crowd of nervous moms and dads. "You'll be testing your blood sugar four times a day and injecting insulin five times a day. In addition, you'll need to log everything you eat and record your blood sugar numbers and the corresponding insulin dose.

"We are going to take you in small groups into the lab," the nurse continued. "We want to make sure you know how to test your blood and determine the right dose of insulin. Oh, and of course, we need to know that you can successfully give yourself a shot, multiple times in the next twenty-four hours."

My mom looked very nervous. I saw her glancing at the exit sign when their names were called for the lab demonstration. When all the parents left, the mood was considerably lighter. The dozen teenagers moved up to the front rows and talked about how their parents would manage the challenge.

"My mother is needle phobic," said one of the guys. "I guarantee you she will not be able to give herself a shot. She can't even look when I inject insulin."

The group laughed.

"This is going to be interesting," said another girl with dark eyeliner and a small tattoo on her wrist. "Now they can see how diabetes sucks."

The afternoon featured separate seminars for the teens and their parents. It was much more interesting to talk about managing diabetes as a member of the football team or the marching band or at prom. It felt good to be in the majority. I realized how tough it was to be the only one with diabetes in my grade of five hundred students.

That night, my parents and I went out to eat at a nearby steak house. After we ordered, my mom pulled out the blood sugar meters and strips. Dad quickly pricked his finger and produced a drop of blood for the glucose meter. Mom tried to be relaxed and casual, but she was taking her time poking her finger.

"Ouch, that hurts," she said. Squeezing hard to get a drop, she managed to get a blood sugar reading. "Are we going to give ourselves a shot right here at the table?" Mom asked.

I laughed. "Where else are you planning to do it? You want to go out to the car or into the bathroom?" They calculated their dose of insulin and drew up the corresponding number of units of saline solution into a needle.

"That didn't hurt as much as I thought it would," Mom said. "But it takes so much time."

"You get used to it," I replied. "I can test my blood and inject the insulin in less than a minute."

"Wow," said Dad. "That is impressive."

It felt good to hear them compliment me for following the insulin regime day after day after day with almost no complaints. Back at the hotel, we were getting ready for bed. Mom was already curled up reading her book.

"Mom, have you tested your blood sugar tonight?" I asked.

"Quinn, I'm so tired. It's been a long day. I've already done it once today."

"I wish I could take a night off from diabetes," I said. "You've had diabetes for nine hours and you're already giving up." My eyes filled with tears.

Mom jumped out of bed and came over to hug me.

"I'm proud of you, Quinn. Your dad and I would trade places with you in a minute if we could. But I would have to really practice with those needles," she said. "This day has been a big eye-opener for us."

They promised they would always do everything in their power to support Will and me living the best life despite having diabetes. And they've kept their word. My parents have allowed us to push the limits.

It wasn't easy but they were not going to limit my life.

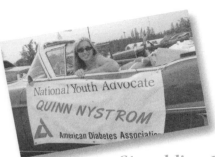

National Youth Advocate
QUINN NYSTROM
American Diabetes Association

CHAPTER 8
Stumbling Blocks to Stepping Stones

I returned to school in the fall as an eighth grader with a whole new attitude. Diabetes was no longer a big deal for me. If it's a big deal for you, that's your problem. I guess I had moved into my militant phase. If somebody wanted to make fun about my diabetes, I would respond. "My pancreas doesn't work. What's your problem?" End of conversation.

I continued with all the activities I loved, including student council, and was an enthusiastic member of the tennis, golf, and cross-country ski teams. One of my favorite activities was figure skating and I took lessons every week.

My parents made it clear that I could have as much independence as I wanted if I was willing to be responsible about my diabetes. The alternative—my parents following me around—was so dreadful that I took full control of managing my disease. I checked my blood sugar by poking my finger and producing a drop of blood. The blood went onto a small strip that was pushed into a palm-sized device that would produce a blood sugar number. Once I knew my blood sugar level, I had a scale to figure out how much insulin I needed. I quickly drew the insulin into the needle and injected it to lower my blood sugar to a target level.

Despite my former life as a confirmed needle phobic, I thought I was doing quite well. It really comes down to this—take multiple shots of insulin a day or die. It's amazing what you can get used to.

Each summer I would meet my friend Nicole at Camp Needlepoint. We'd kept in touch the rest of the year by long phone calls narrating each other's stories of our drama-filled middle-school lives. It was great to have a close friend with diabetes to talk things over with.

It felt like a homecoming to be back at camp, seeing old friends and meeting new ones. At Needlepoint, everyone gathered at the flagpole after lunch for announcements. One day, Becky, the camp director, told us there was a very special speaker in camp. She introduced Clare Rosenfeld, the American Diabetes Association's national youth advocate. One young person from across the country was chosen each year to be the face of diabetes and represent the organization.

Clare was fourteen years old, just like me. She had frizzy, brown hair and was from the West Coast. She talked about her national crusade to find a cure for diabetes. I was mesmerized. "Join the fight," Clare stated. "You can make a difference."

Right then, I decided that I wanted to apply to be the next national youth advocate. If Clare could do it, so could I. When Will was diagnosed with diabetes at five years old, I told him I would do anything I could to find a cure. I thought that meant collecting donations in the neighborhood. I had no idea that a young person could be a national spokesperson for the cause.

I returned home and researched the application process through the American Diabetes Association. I worked hard getting recommendation letters and wrote an essay about my passion for diabetes advocacy. Two months later, I received a letter informing me I had not been chosen. I was insulted when I was passed over for an eleven-year-old boy!

But diabetes had taught me not to give up. The next year, I worked hard to hone my speaking skills. I shared my story of living with diabetes, and my commitment to help find a cure for the disease in classrooms around the school district. I visited young children in the hospital who had just been diagnosed with diabetes and tried to encourage them. I joined a monthly diabetes support group and redoubled my efforts to raise money for the cause.

On March 17, 2002, the exact date of my three-year anniversary with diabetes, I got the call that I had been chosen as the national youth advocate for the American Diabetes Association. Within a month, I was flying to Washington, DC, to train for the role. My first speech was in front of a packed auditorium of American Diabetes Association staff members. I was sixteen years old and didn't know enough to be nervous. I was wearing a pink turtleneck sweater and a gray skirt with my long, dark-blond hair in a ponytail. I was hoping it would pass for a teenage version of business casual. I talked about my little brother and his courage and determination. I spoke of my journey with diabetes. When I finished, they broke into enthusiastic applause. Carlea Bauman, the advocacy chairperson for the American Diabetes Association and my handler for the next year, said I had done a great job.

"You are going to be great, Quinn," she told me. "Just be yourself."

The next day was media training and then a visit to the United States Congress to meet with the United States senators from Minnesota. I really had to pinch myself. I couldn't believe these important people would take the time to listen to a teenager from a small town in Minnesota. Senator Paul Wellstone came out of a hearing to visit with me. I shared my story of living with diabetes and my commitment to find a cure. He listened carefully and then told me of the medical condition he lived with, multiple sclerosis. Senator Wellstone promised he would do what he could to support funding for diabetes.

Wow, I thought. It's hard to imagine I've been given this incredible opportunity.

My year as the national youth advocate was a whirlwind. I traveled across the country to convention halls, camps, schools, and was even invited to the White House. I met lots of heroes with diabetes. Nicole Johnson, the first Miss America to have a chronic disease, was wearing her insulin pump when she was crowned. Gary Hall Jr., the fastest swimmer in the world with a chest full of Olympic gold medals to prove it, had all the right stuff except for his faulty pancreas. It was hard to imagine all these celebrities who were living life large despite diabetes. Talk about role models. I got the message. Diabetes was not an excuse any-more. It would only limit me if I let it.

In June of 2002, our family flew to San Francisco for the annual American Diabetes Association's Scientific Sessions. It was my formal introduction as the new national youth advocate. In front of a packed convention hall, I was introduced by Miss America 1999, Nicole John-son. It was hard to imagine that only months before I was just a small town girl living a very normal life and now I was in San Francisco on a stage and hearing enthusiastic applause after I got done speaking.

I wished I could trade outfits with Nicole. She was wearing a glam-orous dark jacket and skirt with sky-high heels. I was the high-school sophomore in a lime-green cardigan sweater and a black A-line skirt. When I got off the stage I told my mom we had to go shopping immedi-ately. The big banquet was that night and I was not going in the dumb dress I had brought along. She agreed and we found an ebony dress scattered with sequins for the black-tie event.

The next morning, my second official day on the job, Carlea Bauman grabbed me in between conference sessions. "They want you to have lunch with the secretary of Health and Human Services, Tommy Thompson."

"What am I supposed to say?"

"Just be yourself," said Carlea. "You may only have two minutes to tell your story. It's a great opportunity for our organization. Don't worry. You're going to be great."

Just before noon, I was passed off to Secretary Thompson's han-dlers and whisked away through corridors to a beautiful room set for lunch. Four adults were already sitting at the table, Secretary Thompson, his assistant and two bigwigs from the American Diabetes Association. There was one empty chair. As I took my seat, they introduced them-selves and welcomed me as the new national youth advocate. I smiled and said hello, while my mind was spinning. How in the world did I wind up here? They were all so gracious and wanted to hear my story while we ate lunch. I could hardly swallow as I talked about my little brother and then my own diagnosis. I told of my commitment to find a cure and then I asked for Thompson's help.

There were lighter moments as well. Secretary Thompson was the former governor of Wisconsin and served when Jesse Ventura, a former professional wrestler, was the governor of Minnesota. I confessed that one of my favorite T-shirts from the Minnesota state fair proclaimed, "My governor can beat up your governor." We had a good laugh together.

Secretary Thompson later said in his speech that day, "I have no intention of declaring victory until a victory is won. I will not accept such a thing as a "tolerable" incidence of diabetes. I will not stand for an "acceptable" number of Americans dead or maimed from this disease. I will not rest while we can still research more - educate more - and treat more Americans." I walked away with such an incredible respect for this man and the critical work he has done for diabetes. I was honored to be invited to the luncheon that day.

I was completely stunned when he said, "And I'd like to recognize Miss Quinn Nystrom your National Youth Advocate. Quinn, when I was 16, my ambition was to be prominent in Wisconsin. You're already prominent throughout America. Well done." I would have fallen off my chair if my Mom hadn't propped me up.

I learned an important lesson that day. It doesn't matter how old you are or who you are. Even if you are a sixteen-year-old, small-town girl, people will listen if you are willing to tell your personal story with honesty and passion.

I returned to the convention and met many more people with the American Diabetes Association. They welcomed me as the new youth advocate and asked me to visit their state during my year. Later that afternoon, Secretary Thompson's assistant caught up to me. Brent, who had been at the luncheon, asked me what I was doing next weekend. My mind was whirling. Was he asking me on a date?

"I have a lake party with a bunch of my friends," I replied, trying to be cool and casual. "Why?"

"Secretary Thompson was so impressed with you that he is wondering if you would be his guest at the White House for the launch of President George W. Bush's health and fitness campaign," Brent explained. "Can you be there?"

I was a very average student with a very average life. How did this all happen? It was almost beyond my imagination. My parents were as shocked as I was.

The next week I was on the south lawn of the White House as the president launched his health initiative. My dad came along and was even more excited than I was. He could recite the United States presidents in order and their years of service. When we were in elementary school, our family visited Washington, DC, to see all the sights. One of the highlights was taking a tour of the White House, after waiting in a long line to get tickets and then shuffling through with a big group of tourists.

This time was so different. We presented ourselves at a special entrance where we were welcomed and issued identification badges. Wearing our red Diabetes Advocate shirts, we joined Miss America, Nicole Johnson, and the vice-president of the American Diabetes Association.

It was incredible to see the president of the United States and his wife, Laura Bush, pledge their commitment to help prevent type 2 diabetes. President Bush's fitness campaign encouraged everybody to exercise thirty minutes a day, three times a week. A study by the Diabetes Prevention Program, sponsored by the National Institutes of Health, showed that people at risk for type 2 diabetes can, "prevent or delay the onset of the disease by losing 5 to 7 percent of their body weight through increased physical activity and a reduced fat and lower calorie diet."

The south lawn was packed with celebrities. My brothers were so jealous because the entire Washington Redskins football team was there as well as Alan Houston, a basketball player for the New York Knicks, and Dot Richardson, a two-time Olympic gold medalist for the US softball team. I even said "Hi" to Al Roker from the Today Show. The only disappointment was the rose garden, which was strangely missing roses.

Diabetes was the worst thing that ever happened to me. But it was also turning out to be the best thing that ever happened to me. My year as the national youth advocate showed me people can make a difference if they are willing to commit themselves to the cause.

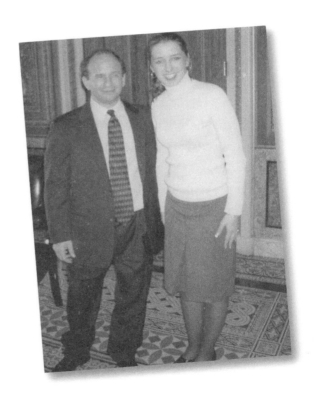

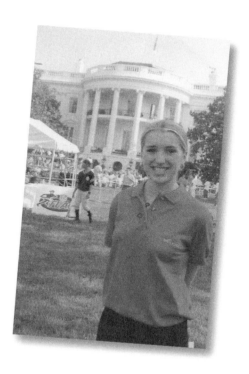

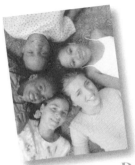

CHAPTER 9
Dateline Diabetes Camps

The best part of my year as national youth advocate was traveling to diabetes camps across the country. It was hard to believe that just three years before, my mom had to force me to attend Camp Needlepoint, and now I was being introduced as the guest speaker! At each camp I would share my story and encourage them to join the fight to find a cure for diabetes. At the end of the speech, I would ask for questions. The campers took me completely by surprise. I thought they would ask me "get to know you" questions. Instead, they wanted answers on real life issues that I too struggled with. I was so impressed by their commitment and courage. I loved their questions and was so happy and honored that they valued my opinions. That was a rarity in my house with two brothers who never listened to what I had to say.

Here are some of my online journal entries from the summer diabetes camp tour.

July 2, 2002—Camp Clara Barton, North Oxford, Massachusetts

Kids are interested in diabetes! Kids are interested in a cure! Camp Clara Barton was the first stop on my tour of diabetes summer camps. I'm traveling around the country, talking to campers about diabetes advocacy and getting involved in the fight for a cure.

What a warm welcome I received (and I'm not just talking about the ninety-degree temperature!). After a tour of the camp (nice cabins, no port-a-potties!), I talked to the campers about the obstacles I have faced in my life with diabetes and my crusade to find a cure. I invited them to join the fight and become diabetes advocates. You don't have to wait until you're a grown-up. I have found out that people will listen to us if we are willing to speak up. Later in the day, I joined a couple of cabins for a bonfire dinner.

I ended the day by visiting Camp Joslin (Clara Barton's brother camp). One of the counselors was a guy I met in Washington, DC, at the Call to Congress: Conquer Diabetes in May. Jake gave me the grand tour and introduced me to the campers. It was so scorching hot I ended up jumping in the lake in my clothes. (Jake gave me a Camp Joslin T-shirt to change into. It's a cute shirt. Most important, it was dry. I'm wearing it as I write this.) I can't believe how much fun today was! I love summer camps! These are my types of people!

July 17, 2002—Camp Conrad-Chinnock, near Los Angeles, California

I feel like a traveling salesman. My second camp visit took me all the way across the country to California. Hollywood, here we come! Even though this camp is thousands of miles away from the last camp, the kids are concerned about the same things.

"How do I deal with diabetes?"

"Should I tell people I have diabetes or keep it a secret?"

"When will they find a cure?"

Those of us with diabetes all wrestle with the same issues. That's the great thing about going to a diabetes camp. For the first time, you get to be in a crowd of kids who all have to monitor their blood glucose levels many times a day and count carbohydrates. It's great to know you are not the only one living with it.

My trip to Conrad-Chinnock was one I won't forget. I've never been on top of a mountain before. This camp sits seven thousand feet up in the California Mountains. It was a long and winding road up here—I thought I was going to throw up. The air was sweet with the smell of pine trees. I was impressed that there were no mosquitoes (which are the state "bird" of Minnesota!). After a tour of the camp, I spoke to 120 campers and sixty staff members. The kids were really interested in my position as national youth advocate and how they can get involved. This mountaintop experience will be unforgettable.

July 18–20, 2002—Friends for Life Conference, Pasadena, California

Can you imagine three hotels full of kids with diabetes, and their families? Throw in great seminars and discussion groups, celebrities, a day at Universal Studios, and even a teen dance and you have the annual Friends for Life Conference.

My dad and younger brother, Will, came along. We had the best time. A highlight for us was meeting Gary Hall Jr., the Olympic gold medalist swimmer. I remember watching him compete during the Olympics and cheering him on from our family room in northern Minnesota. When Gary was diagnosed with diabetes, his doctor told him his competitive swimming career was over. He found a new doctor and the rest is history. When it was time for questions and answers, my little brother shot his arm up. "Gary, did you wear your gold medal when you got married?" How embarrassing. Gary just laughed and said it would have been a good idea but no, he didn't. For the rest of the conference, Gary called Will "Spanky" every time he saw him. Not all heroes have a functioning pancreas. Go, Gary, go.

July 23, 2002—Camp Earthworks, Springfield, Missouri

What a sweet welcome when I arrived at Camp Earthworks. A crowd of young campers greeted me with a big "Welcome Quinn" sign and huge smiles. The campers were the youngest I have met so far. They were good listeners and had some great questions for me. They told me about their struggles with diabetes. One little girl with a blond ponytail remembered the day she was diagnosed and went to the hospital. She said her mom and dad both cried and she didn't understand why. It broke my heart.

We talked about our heroes. There is a camp full of them in Springfield. These kids, as young as kindergarteners, monitor their blood, inject insulin, and keep right on going. They were interested in seeing my in-

sulin pump and wanted to hear about my younger brother, Will, who also has diabetes. I told them that we sometimes compete with each other to see who has a better blood sugar reading or who can get their results fastest.

After our talk, we headed for the swimming pool. It was hot out and the water was nice and cool. I felt like a jungle gym because the kids climbed all over me in the pool. At this camp, the brothers, sisters, and friends of kids with diabetes are invited along. It's a great opportunity for everybody to learn more about diabetes. I carefully rolled up the "Welcome Quinn" poster with their signatures. I'm going to put it on my bedroom door to help me remember that kids all over the country are waiting and hoping and praying for a cure for diabetes.

July 29, 2002—Camp Shawnee, Kansas City, Missouri

On one sunny, humid day outside Kansas City, my mom and I pulled up in our rented PT Cruiser to Camp Discovery. We were greeted by a teenage guy with reddish hair and freckles sprinkled across his face. "Hi, I'm Matt," he said. "This is my favorite week of the year. When I get home from camp, I start the countdown for the next year."

Now that's a commitment. Those of us with diabetes all wrestle with the same issues. That's the great thing about going to a diabetes camp. For the first time, you get to be in a crowd of kids who all have to monitor their blood glucose levels many times a day and count carbs. You get to see kids and counselors who don't let the disease get in the way of living.

Camp Shawnee is set among the rolling hills of Missouri. These kids must feel like mountain goats as they go from their cabins to the dining hall and around to all of their activities. The camp director, Joby Jobson, was the national youth spokesman for the ADA when he was younger. It was an earlier version of the national youth advocate program. Joby told me what a wonderful experience he had with the ADA leadership program. Not only did he make friends from around the country, he met his future wife! Emily was the national youth spokesperson the year after Joby. Now that's a diabetes power couple!

August 9, 2002—Camp Fun in the Sun, Rathdrum, Idaho

What an honor to visit the home camp of the legendary Washington State teen advocates. These guys literally wrote the book on teen advocacy. In fact, during my camp visits, I've been handing out the Teen Advocacy Manual they wrote to show kids how to put together a teen diabetes advocacy group in their own hometowns.

I'm in awe of the progress they've made in the last year fighting for the rights of those living with diabetes. Thanks to the Washington teen advocates, the state legislature passed laws to allow kids with diabetes to receive adequate care for their diabetes while in school.

This was my first diabetes teen camp and it was nonstop fun. Dances, karaoke, skit night, and lots of time to hang out and talk. I got in on some water relay races. It was wild! We divided into teams and raced canoes on a course on Lake Coeur d'Alene.

When they heard I was from Minnesota, the land of ten thousand lakes, they insisted I captain the canoe. Despite me, our team won. The guys and girls were so friendly and made me feel a part of things. We talked about how you can make a difference in your community and why we don't have to be embarrassed or ashamed because we have diabetes. So my pancreas doesn't work, so what? Get over it and get on with it.

August 16, 2002—Camp Setebaid, Shickshinny, Pennsylvania

The question that most surprised me while I was visiting diabetes summer camps happened at Camp Setebaid in Shickshinny, Pennsylvania. It was a hot, humid night and all the campers were crowded in the dining hall after supper for my presentation. I told them about being diagnosed with diabetes and committing to find a cure. I shared my camp travels and stories about the cool kids with diabetes I met from coast to coast. Before I finished speaking, a young boy, maybe ten years old, stuck his arm as high as he could in the air.

He was soft-spoken but very earnest. "Do you enjoy having diabetes?" I was so taken aback by his question but my answer was swift and strong.

"Do I enjoy having diabetes? Absolutely not!" I responded. "Diabetes is a disease that you can never take a vacation from, not even for a day. You're constantly thinking about your blood sugar every minute of every day. I hate having diabetes."

I looked around the packed room filled with campers and counselors living with diabetes. "Being diagnosed with diabetes was the worst day of my life," I continued. "I didn't think I would be able to live with diabetes. But I didn't have a choice and neither do you. Eventually I realized my only choice was how I was going to live."

Long after I left Shickshinny, I was still thinking about that boy's question. Have I gone overboard? Am I trying to glamorize diabetes? I hope not. As a speaker, I want to be realistic about the challenges of living with diabetes. But I also want to encourage other diabetics to stand up and be counted. Join our fight to find a cure for diabetes. Together, we can do it. I wish I knew what that little boy's name was. I still think of him.

At twenty-seven years of age, I still visit diabetes camps as a member of the America Diabetes Association's Minnesota Community Leadership Board. Every August we meet at Camp Needlepoint in Hudson, Wisconsin. When I visited Camp Needlepoint in 2013, an eight-year-old camper was asked to share his camp experiences. Jordan was asked how many kids in his school have diabetes. He answered quietly, "I think I'm the only one in the world with diabetes." When asked what made Camp Needlepoint different from school, he got excited. "It's like a million people here have diabetes!" It was the first place Jordan felt normal. At Needlepoint, he was in the majority and loving every minute of it. It brought tears to my eyes because I knew exactly how he felt.

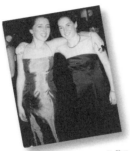

CHAPTER 10
If I Kiss You Will I Get Diabetes?

My dating life took a nosedive before it could even take off. When I was diagnosed with diabetes, I withdrew from a lot of relationships. I didn't want to share what was really going on in my life. My motto was to reject before I could be rejected. I had a close group of girlfriends who were supportive, but I didn't want to venture into the dating scene. When I was in high school, when school dances were the highlights of the social calendar, I always had a date but never a boyfriend.

At Christmas Ball, held at a nearby resort, my dear friend Stina and I were doubling with a pair of exchange students from our high school. My Spaniard, Alberto, was tall, dark, and handsome. I loved my purple taffeta gown and sophisticated updo. Stina, who was going with a Swede, wore a navy strapless dress that showed off her toned swimmer's shoulders. Because our foreign exchange student dates didn't have cars or driver's licenses, Stina drove the four of us to the dance in her parents' blue Suburban.

In Brainerd, if you weren't a steady couple, you danced with lots of different guys during the evening. Our dates gravitated to their fellow international students and Stina and I joined other friends. Christmas Ball was the swankiest dance of the year, because it wasn't held in the school gym. There were still lots of parent-chaperones and mandatory Breathalyzer tests when we arrived at Cragun's Resort on Gull Lake. The sports center was transformed with white twinkle lights and loud music booming from speakers in the DJ booth.

I was hoping to meet up with Sean. We were good friends and had a lot in common. We were involved in student government and community causes. Everybody liked Sean, even my parents. I had a crush on him. He found me in the crowd and we headed for the dance floor. It was a great night and getting better all the time. When the music slowed down, Sean pulled me close for a slow dance. When he leaned in for our first kiss, my heart literally skipped a beat and butterflies soared. And then he paused.

"If I kiss you, will I get diabetes?" Sean asked.

Sharp stab in my heart. Butterflies dead.

"Absolutely not!" I said. "Do you think diabetes is contagious?"

"I don't know." Sean looked miserable. "There is so much talk about AIDS and how it spreads, I just wanted to make sure. I want to kiss you, but I don't want to get diabetes."

Tears sprang to my eyes. I whirled away from him and ran from the dance floor. I wanted to go home. The bathroom was jammed with girls redoing their hair and putting on more makeup. I walked outside to compose myself, but I had to return quickly because the temperatures were below zero on that frigid night in December.

I sat down at a table with my girlfriends and tried to act normal, but my mind was spinning. Sean was a sweet guy, and smart. Does everybody think diabetes is contagious? Maybe I should hang a large bell around my neck and go around yelling "Unclean, unclean..." like Typhoid Mary.

I didn't think things could get any worse. But at the end of the night, I saw Sean on the dance floor kissing Mary, a tall girl with long, curly hair and an unbroken string of straight As. What does she have that I don't? I thought. Oh, that's right. She doesn't have a disease that he might catch on the dance floor.

That night, I felt like my love life was over before it really got started. Maybe everybody thinks I'm contagious. I was frustrated and heartbroken. I wanted to give up.

Living with diabetes all these years, people ask the oddest questions. At first I was offended and hurt like when Sean thought the disease was contagious. But I had to be honest with myself. What did I know about diabetes before Will was diagnosed? Just about nothing. I thought he would have to stay in the hospital and wouldn't be able to come back home.

My attitude changed and I was grateful for people who would ask questions (but not right before a kiss!). If I didn't take the opportunity to educate others about diabetes, I had myself to blame for their ignorance. As I got older, I stopped hiding my diabetes. I didn't flaunt it, I just went about my business.

P.S. The broken romance with Sean was for the best. He became a priest and lives in Ireland. I'm in Minnesota and still looking for love!

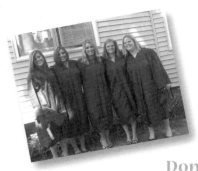

CHAPTER 11
Don't Forget the Insulin

Hallelujah. I made it through high school. Check. Now on to the big adventure—college. After visiting a handful of schools, I chose a college two hours away from my home: Concordia College in Moorhead, Minnesota. It was far enough that my parents wouldn't drop in, but close enough to drive home for the weekend.

College is a new adjustment for everyone. New people, new places, serious studying, and no parents. I couldn't wait. But I was anxious about navigating this new chapter in my life with type 1 diabetes. Along with big plastic totes full of clothes and shoes and books and stuff, I had to pack insulin, needles, pump supplies, blood glucose meters, and boxes of test strips, glucose tablets, etc.

I was a wreck. I had all the standard fears about living with a stranger in a very small room. Did I have to tell her I had diabetes? If I didn't and she found a stash of needles, she might think I was a heroin addict. At least then, she would be relieved I was only a diabetic. Okay, so I'll tell her. "Hi, I'm Quinn. I'm a diabetic." How awkward would that be? Worse yet, she might want to change rooms right away, too nervous to room with a disease condition. Why did I sometimes revert to my thirteen-year-old self? If only I didn't have diabetes. College and life would be so much easier.

Dad turned onto the Concordia campus and pulled up in front of my four-story, brick dormitory, Park Region. A steady stream of students, dressed in the school's colors, gold and maroon, staggered in under loads of cardboard boxes passing a steady stream of people coming out with empty hands. We joined the throng, climbing up to the fourth floor. I was so nervous I could hardly swallow. Every time I caught Mom's eye, she flashed a big smile. I got the message. "Don't worry, Quinn. This is going to be great. You're going to be fine."

"Yeah, Mom. Easy for you to say as you get back into the Jeep with Dad and head home to Brainerd."

Mom and I had talked about how and when I should tell my roommate about my diabetes. I thought I should keep it under wraps for a few weeks, until we knew each other. Then she would realize it wasn't a big deal. My mom suggested it might be better to get it over with.

"It's not a big thing for you, Quinn," she said. "It shouldn't be any big thing for her either. Just tell her and move on."

It sounded logical at the time, but when the moment arrived, my courage had evaporated. I felt like the Lion in the *Wizard of Oz* when the Great Oz demanded that Lion retrieve the broom that belonged to the Wicked Witch. Remember how he ran straight down the aisle away from the wizard and jumped out the window? That's how I felt. And it was a long way down from the fourth floor.

When we got to room 407, my new roommate and her family were already there unpacking.

"Hi, you must be Meghan," I said. She had straight, dark hair, big, brown eyes, and a quick smile.

"Hey, Quinn! It's nice to meet you."

We went around the room introducing our families.

"Is the refrigerator yours?" I asked. "Can I keep my insulin in there? I have type 1 diabetes."

"Sure," Meghan replied. "I have asthma so I totally get it."

That went well, I thought to myself. Maybe this is going to work out.

College was fun and stressful and hard and fun. It was like that for me and everyone else. Diabetes wasn't such a big deal. I was lucky that I had five years under my belt of living with the disease. Late nights and marathon study sessions were a challenge, but it wasn't that bad.

Meghan and I were good roommates. We each had a group of friends and different interests, but we got along well. She was a nursing major, so having a roommate with diabetes was no big deal. She thought it was a bonus.

The following year, another roommate wasn't so empathetic. One night I couldn't get my blood sugars under control. I injected extra insulin but it wasn't working. I was dehydrated and was feeling worse and worse. It was late and the first time I was away from my family while experiencing a health crisis.

"I'm so frustrated with my diabetes. I don't know what to do."

My roommate, Kim, responded softly, "Well, do you think you should go to the hospital?"

"I don't know what to do. Things have just gotten worse, so I guess maybe I should."

I was relieved when Kim agreed with my decision and said she would be happy to drive me to the emergency room.

I was grateful for her kindness and care. After checking all my levels, giving me insulin, and rehydrating through an IV, they sent me home.

Unfortunately, a couple days later, I heard from my friends that she had told people I had faked the whole thing for attention. I was crushed. It was the first time I had ever been to the hospital for anything diabetes related. It hurt that someone I considered a close friend had betrayed me. Why would she do that? If she really knew me, she would understand that the last thing I would want was to bring attention to my disease.

Kim knew I had diabetes but never acknowledged it. She was perfect with the perfect boyfriend, perfect blond hair, and perfect designer clothes. Everything in her life seemed together. She must have been horrified to live with a roommate who was so far from perfect. I never again mentioned my diabetes and made sure she didn't see any evidence of it.

Later in the year, I was struggling to put in a new pump infusion site. Instead of using needles to deliver insulin multiple times a day, I had graduated to a continuous insulin pump. I inserted an infusion set under the skin and then my Medtronic insulin pump released insulin around the clock. When I ate and needed extra insulin, I could push a button to deliver extra insulin. The pump site had to be moved every couple of days and I was having a terrible time trying to put it on the far side of my hip. I had tried four times and the needle kept bending back into my skin. Tears welled in my eyes.

Kim walked through the door. I looked like a hot mess—tubing, insulin vials, and needles were strewn all around me.

"Could you please help me? I asked. "I'm having the hardest time today inserting this set correctly. I just can't get it in."

She looked at me and the paraphernalia. Shaking her head, she said, "That's gross." Kim turned around and walked out of the room.

Sitting on my cranberry futon with my head in my hands, tears streamed down my face.

I cannot do this, I told myself. I'm through. It's too hard. I hate this.

After a good cry, I considered the alternatives. I could forget about the insulin and die, or figure it out. I splashed my face with cold water, looked in the mirror and said, "You can do this. You know you can."

And I did.

After sophomore year, I decided to transfer to Hope College in Holland, Michigan. It was my original choice for college, but I was nervous about being so far away from home. I was looking forward to a fresh start. I met wonderful friends whom I could be myself with. Casi, Beth, Kristen, Jordyn, and Emily made me feel welcome. They didn't care about diabetes. They cared about each other and me. They were there when I landed a dream internship in New York City and then when I found out the devastating breast cancer diagnosis of my dear Grandma Ruth. They were there in the good times and bad. Most important, they helped me develop a sense of humor about diabetes.

One day we were arguing about the utility bills. Instead of splitting it evenly, I suggested we pay based on our utility use. Kristen ran a window air conditioner constantly to keep her bedroom ice cold and Casi had a heated waterbed.

Without missing a beat, my sassy southern roommate, Casi, said, "If we're paying more, so should you. How much electricity does it take to run your insulin pump?"

I responded with a straight face, "Casi, I'm battery operated." We all fell to the floor laughing.

These girls asked if they could test their blood sugar so they would know what it felt like. They were curious about diabetes and how it felt to live with it. We were able to be honest about the hard things in our lives. I had diabetes, but each of them struggled in other ways. I can't tell you what it felt like to have these beautiful, loyal, caring friends. Years later we still carry each other's burdens and celebrate the joys. It felt great to be judged by my *heart* rather than my pancreas.

CHAPTER 12
Purpose and Passion

The day Will was diagnosed with diabetes was the day I realized what I wanted to be when I grew up. I was ten years old and I was going to find the cure for this horrible disease that had blown up his life and dreams. Unlike other childhood dreams, I never wavered in my commitment. I was going to spend my life attempting to find a cure. I pictured myself in a white lab coat surrounded by test tubes.

I would do it.

Years later, in high school chemistry, I had to face the facts. I was not the scientific type. I was never going to discover the cure for diabetes. It was a big blow. My commitment never wavered, but I had to be realistic. If I couldn't be a scientist, how was I going to help find a cure? Instead, I focused on my work with the American Diabetes Association. As the youth advocate, I did not require scientific talent. Telling my story helped raise awareness of the disease and the desperately needed funding to find a cure.

What a relief! Good-bye chemistry, hello communications. I had the same goal but a new focus. I would develop my communication skills to lobby for legislation to help fund a cure and provide help for the twenty-five million Americans living with diabetes. In college, I majored in public relations and political science with the hope of a career in diabetes advocacy.

Diabetes advocacy has taken many paths in my life. Sometimes I have the opportunity to address large gatherings. Other times I have the privilege to deliver the message to an individual. When I was in college, I got a call from my mom telling me about a young girl who had just been diagnosed with diabetes. Jen was thirteen years old—the same age I was when I had been diagnosed. Jen's mom called my mother and said her daughter was really struggling. In a small town, our family served as a diabetes hotline. When Will was diagnosed, my parents were so grateful for the support of other families with children living with diabetes. They were a source of encouragement and education and hope. Mom had a long conversation with Jen's mom and talked about my own trials when I was diagnosed at age thirteen. Then she called me and asked if I would reach out to Jen.

I first sent an e-mail to Jen introducing myself. The words didn't come as easily as I thought they would. I wanted to be positive and a good role model. How helpful would it be to tell her about the kids who teased me, my failure to accept the terms of the illness, and the pain of those years? I just asked her if she wanted to get together and talk. Jen responded right away and wondered how soon we could get together.

We met up a few weeks later during my December college break. I remember thinking that Jen's thick, dark eye makeup acted like a mask to hide her vulnerability. She kept her eyes on her hot chocolate as we spoke. I had to lean forward to hear what she said.

"My mom blames my issues on my diabetes."

"Do you agree with her?"

"Yes. I guess," she mumbled.

My heart broke as I remembered my painful journey through seventh grade with diabetes. Going back to those dark days is something I avoid. But I had been down the same road Jen was walking, and I wanted to let her know about my hurdles that I had worked hard to overcome. My heart broke when Jen pulled up the sleeves of her woolen coat to show the fresh red slashes on her arms. She confessed that she had been self-mutilating, cutting herself on her arms and legs, because the physical pain somehow eased the inner pain she was feeling.

After our first meeting, Jen and I e-mailed back and forth. Every couple of months, I would meet her for lunch and talk about how we were coping with diabetes. A year later, Jen decided to check into a hospital to get help for her emotional issues.

I had lunch with her a year later. She is a healthy, happy young woman. We talked about boys, school, and boys. Jen still has diabetes and so do I, but the disease cannot determine the quality of our lives unless we let it.

A chronic disease is a marathon rather than a sprint. It's exhausting. There is no end in sight for those who live with diabetes. When Will was diagnosed, we were sure that a cure would be found before he went to high school. Now he's finishing college and we are still waiting for the miracle.

There are days when I wake up and am still upset about having diabetes almost fifteen years after my diagnosis. I feel sorry for myself and I'm exhausted. Some have called it "diabetes burnout." When I have one of these days I wonder, why can't I get over it and accept this part of my life?

It helps for me to turn away from the disease and think about the many blessings in my life. I am surrounded by a loving family and wonderful friends. I have a purpose and a passion that gives life meaning. Diabetes destroyed my pancreas, but everything else still works. Life is good. And I am not just a chronic illness.

I was waitressing at a restaurant in college and my insulin pump started beeping. I had forgotten to switch the alert to vibrate before I began work. I am not ashamed of having diabetes, but never make a big deal about it. What is the point of announcing you have an incurable illness? I had just started working at Grizzly's and wanted to fit in with the rest of the staff.

"Do you have low blood sugar or something?" asked one of the servers.

I was stunned that he had figured out that the beep was from an insulin pump.

"How did you guess?" I said.

"I've had type 1 diabetes for several years now and used to be on the pump myself. Not my thing though. I just do shots now," he answered.

"Cool."

A couple weeks later there was a diabetes event in our community and I asked my coworker, "Would you be interested in volunteering at the annual Walk for Diabetes?"

"No thanks. Not my thing," he replied.

"Okay," I said. "But you have diabetes. Aren't you interested in helping to find a cure?"

"Quinn, the way I look at it is that I live with this disease twenty-four-seven and I'm just plain burned out from it." He shook his head like a tired, old man. "It's that simple."

Some people can't or won't accept the terms of the illness. Sometimes I feel the same way. There will never be a cure for diabetes. Will and I will grow old and we will still be relying on insulin day after day to stay alive. Thankfully, those days of despair don't happen too often. We can't give up on finding a cure. Just imagine if all twenty-five million diabetics stood up against this disease and fought for a cure? We would be unstoppable. I'm no scientist, but I know we would be much closer to a cure and better treatments for diabetes. We cannot give up.

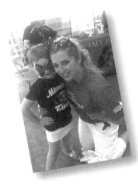

CHAPTER 13
Ignorance Isn't Bliss

Brian worked with me at a pharmaceutical distribution company, my first professional job out of college. He was a great guy. Cute, nice, and single and we had known each other for three years. We were at a national sales meeting and the company hosted a night at the St. Louis Cardinal's baseball game. A group of us decided to grab dinner before the game. As we sat around a big, round table waiting for our food, I put my insulin pump on the table and searched my purse for glucose tabs. I felt a tug on my skin where the pump was attached. I looked up to see Brian, with my pump in his hand.

"What are you doing?" I asked.

"Isn't this a pager?" he replied. "I just want to see what model you have."

"No, it's my insulin pump," I explained. "What the heck do you think the plastic tubing is?"

"I don't know," Brian answered. "I thought it was some kind of leash connected to your belt so you wouldn't lose the pager. Why do you have an insulin pump?"

I told the group I had diabetes. A couple of them already knew. In the end, we all had a good laugh at Brian. A pager? Really? It was 2011. Did they even make pagers anymore? If you are comfortable talking about diabetes, everyone else will be comfortable also.

When I was attending Hope College, I interned with the American Diabetes Association in Michigan. They had asked me to do an interview about diabetes with a local television station. The interview was live and the tape was rolling.

The broadcaster asked some basic questions about diabetes and then out of nowhere commented, "I just have to say this. You just don't look like you have diabetes."

I was flabbergasted by her comment and quickly responded, "What does a diabetic look like?"

I must have caught her off guard because she described a diabetic as "old, overweight, out of shape, and sickly." I couldn't believe she was saying this live on a news program. I quickly corrected her.

"My little brother was diagnosed with diabetes the year before he went to kindergarten. I was thirteen years old when I got it," I explained. "Diabetes affects people of all ages and ethnicities. They look like anyone else—old and young, rich and poor, athletic and sedentary."

The newscaster recovered quickly and confessed she didn't know much about the disease that affects twenty-five million Americans. I helped her and the viewers understand the difference between type 1 and type 2 diabetes and the urgent need for research. There is no need to put someone down because they are misinformed about diabetes. It works much better to educate them. My goal is to find a cure for diabetes, and that requires a groundswell of financial support and research. I'm hoping that newscaster learned a lesson. If she wants to be trustworthy, she has to have the facts.

The general public doesn't know much about diabetes. Our family didn't, until it moved into our house. There are a variety of opinions about diagnosis and treatment even among the medical community. The latest about diabetes today might be totally outdated by tomorrow.

Even in the diabetes world, there are disagreements. Some are significant and some are minor. I get a laugh over the debate of what to call someone who has diabetes. Some health care professionals and members of the diabetes community are trying to replace the term "diabetic." They feel it is more accurate to use the term "a person living with diabetes."

I don't care. Call me whatever you like. But others feel very strongly about it. My dad, a pharmacist, is the kindest guy in the world. He still uses the term "diabetics." It's shorter and easier. In no way is he labeling or negating those living with diabetes. A bigger and more important issue, in my mind, is helping educate the public about the difference between type 1 and type 2. My advice is to save your energy for bigger issues. As Eleanor Roosevelt wrote, "No one can make you feel inferior without your consent."

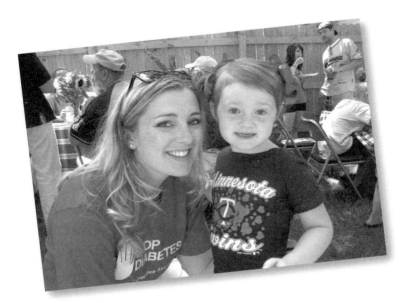

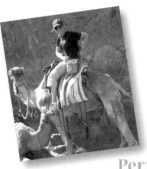

CHAPTER 14
Perfectionists Need Not Apply

Perfectionists need not apply for diabetes. It's an illness that you can never be "perfect" at. Once you get that in your mind, life will be much better. Blood glucose levels are fickle. Some days your blood glucose levels will fluctuate wildly because of stress or a cold. Some nights you go to bed with a perfectly normal blood sugar of 105, but wake up in the middle of the night with a dangerously low reading of 45. This is a disease where you can do everything right but still come up short. Emotions, activity, certain foods, and a hundred other factors can affect blood sugars. Let your friends and family know how frustrating it is so they can encourage you in the dark days. A support system is mandatory for a person living with diabetes.

Imagine taking a test that you studied hard for. You knew all the answers to all the questions. All that's left is to see the big, beautiful A marked on the top of the graded test. But what if it comes back with an F instead? That's what diabetes feels like. Doing everything right and still ending up short of the mark. Knowing that you can't control what you can't control is a relief. It takes the pressure off. Some days having a blood sugar of 200 needs to be celebrated. Other days you can cheer with a blood sugar of 120. Do not live or die by the numbers. Diabetes is all about progress not perfection.

There is much discussion about the "perfect" A1C in the diabetes world. A1C is a test that measures a person's average blood glucose levels over two to three months. It gives you a good idea of how well your diabetes treatment plan is working. The American Diabetes Association likens the A1C to a baseball player's season batting average.

"It tells you about a person's overall success. Neither a single day's blood test results nor a single game's batting record gives the same big picture," according to ADA literature.

The goal for diabetics is to keep their A1C results as close as possible to a person who has a functioning pancreas. It helps avoid the complications that can result from diabetes. So what is the perfect A1C? Always remember that it is a number with a lot of variables.

In my work with diabetes advocacy, I've talked with top endocrinologists across the country about A1Cs. They agree that it doesn't provide the complete measure of health. Someone with an A1C of 6.8 percent (an admirable target) may have dangerously low blood sugars followed by high swings. It looks good on paper, but does not reflect good control of the disease. Ask your doctor for a target goal and then do your best to manage your blood sugars on a daily basis. It's way too easy to beat yourself up if you live by the numbers. I had a low A1C number, but I was struggling with bad hypoglycemic reactions. My doctor suggested it would be healthier for me to stay below 7.5 percent as a type 1 diabetic.

After fifteen years of living with diabetes, I don't obsess about my blood sugars. I remember sitting in the emergency room on a Friday night because my blood sugars would not drop below 300 (in forty-eight hours) because of a bad reaction to prednisone. I *will not, will not, will not* beat myself up over times like that. I will not obsess if A1C fluctuates slightly. I don't think that's healthy. The first thing we have to accept when we're diagnosed with diabetes is that we do not have complete control of our blood sugars. I want people I speak with to know that I'm not perfect, that I'm a regular patient who tries to hit my goals on a daily basis. I don't speak of being the "perfect diabetic," because I don't think that's accurate or possible. Understand and accept that there are some things you can't control. Do your best and move forward. Just keep repeating: progress, not perfection, is the real goal.

I woke up one morning with my insulin pump lying next to me on my bedside table. It was no longer connected to my body. And my continuous glucose monitor was on the floor. I must have pulled them both out sometime during the night. My heart dropped. My mind raced. I live alone, and one of my biggest fears is having a dangerously low blood sugar overnight. I'm afraid I won't wake soon enough to correct a plummeting blood sugar.

That morning, I jumped out of bed to grab my blood glucose meter on the dresser. I pricked my pointer finger with the lancet and squeezed a drop of blood onto the meter. I watched as the machine counted down 5, 4, 3, 2, 1…489. My blood sugar was five times higher than normal and I felt like I had a bad case of the flu, including a terrible headache and a jumpy stomach. Worse yet, my confidence was shaken. How can I control my diabetes if I'm capable of pulling out my pump infusion set in my sleep? What if I hadn't woken? My mind quickly descended into an assortment of dangerous possibilities. Those are the worst diabetes days.

Going back to bed and pulling the covers over my head was not an option. I was scheduled to speak at a Rotary meeting about my journey with diabetes. I was not going to cancel, so I dressed and drove to the event. As a motivational speaker, I try to inspire the audience with an upbeat message. It was hard to admit to others that I was sometimes the "bad diabetic." I blamed myself for low blood sugars and high blood sugars. It was hard to be honest about the struggles because I want to be a good example for others, especially for young people. As I drove along, I felt inadequate. What am I doing? What am I going to say to them?

That morning in Waconia, I was introduced by a lovely woman named Nancy. She spoke of my background as a speaker with the American Diabetes Association. She paused and said, "My mother recently passed away. She lived with diabetes for sixty-five years." Nancy paused again and looked out over the crowd. "It isn't an easy illness to live with. My mother was a survivor."

Instead of my usual speech about my diagnosis at thirteen, being ashamed, getting over it, and then turning stumbling blocks into stepping-stones, Nancy inspired me to be brutally honest. I delivered a raw perspective on what it feels like to be a twenty-five-year-old woman with type 1 diabetes—the good, the bad, and the very ugly.

I concluded the speech with what had happened the past evening. I shared my fears of dying in my sleep because of undetected low blood sugar. I also told them about striving to be perfect, to be an inspiration for others with perfect blood sugars and a perfect life. I didn't want to show any weakness. I admitted that I needed to ask others for help in this difficult journey. When I looked over to Nancy, she was weeping.

She jumped out of her chair and walked to the podium. "Quinn, you have honored my mother's memory today. Thank you." Nancy threw her arms around me and the Rotarians gave a heartfelt round of applause.

I learned an important lesson that day from Nancy. We do each other a disservice when we edit our life story into an impossible string of successes. Perfectionism is not a strength, and vulnerability is not a weakness.

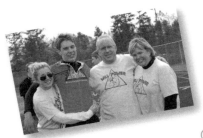

CHAPTER 15
Not All Heroes Wear Capes

When my brother Will was born, he had two sets of parents. I was six and our older brother, Thor, was seven years old. Will was our living, breathing baby doll. I remember passing out blue bubble gum cigars to my kindergarten class the day he was born. But when it came to diabetes years later, I was definitely the baby of the family.

Growing up in the exact same family of five, living in the same house in the same small northern Minnesota town, Will and I also shared a disease. I want to include his perspective as an example of how two people with so much in common react very differently to the same circumstances. Will is still my baby brother, even though he's six feet four inches tall and a senior at Baylor University in Texas. I called him this week on the eve of his 22nd birthday and asked him some questions about his experiences with diabetes.

"Will, do you remember being hospitalized for five days after your diagnosis of type 1 diabetes in December 1996?"

Without missing a beat Will said, "I thought it was really fun. I had a whole wing of the hospital to myself."

I have vivid memories of being in the hospital with Will and my mom, who spent most of her time sobbing, almost uncontrollable with her emotions. My dad, a pharmacist, owned two pharmacies and worked long hours. He would show up in the evening to provide some relief. I was scared to death that Will would never leave the hospital.

"Hey, Quinn, remember Mr. Keller pushing me in a race car up and down the halls? That was a blast," Will recalled. "I had my own Nintendo and didn't have to share with anyone."

While Will greeted his many visitors, Mom received a crash course on diabetes from the nurses. She had to go through a workbook and then answer test questions. The low point was when a nurse told Mom very firmly, "Will won't be able to leave the hospital until you are capable of giving him a shot of insulin." That's when the tears really started to flow.

"I can't. I just can't do it," Mom said over and over again. "I'm afraid of needles."

Dad would come to the hospital after work and the five of us would have dinner together. Will's meals were strictly regulated down to the last french fry. Then Dad, Thor, and I would head home. Will gave a cheerful wave good-bye and Mom managed a wan smile. She slept in a little bed that pulled out from a cabinet next to Will's hospital bed.

Besides remembering lots of gifts and visitors, Will says he doesn't remember much about diabetes. He returned to preschool the next week and got on with his life.

"Diabetes is one of those things that you can't complain about," Will said. "You're stuck with it every day, all day, and if you focus on it, you are screwed. You have to be the person that decides to be positive. You can't say this [expletive deleted] disease sucks, even though it does, 'cause these are the cards that were dealt to me."

It's not often that Will and I have a serious conversation, or at least his half of the conversation. Our pattern goes something like this, "Will, I'm worried about _____."

His typical response, "Hey girl, give me some love...."

I can tell Will is smiling even over the telephone. I can't picture him without the crazy, wide grin that creases his face until his eyes almost disappear.

But now I want him to be serious. I want to know what he really thinks about his life with diabetes.

"The truth is, Quinn, bad things happen to everyone. I think I have a great life even if my pancreas doesn't work," Will responds. "What else do you want to know?"

Sometimes I get frustrated with Will. I want him to join me in the fight against diabetes. In junior high, I started serious fundraising for diabetes and I assumed Will would be with me. He wasn't interested and finally told me to stop pushing him.

"If I'm going to go around the neighborhood asking for donations, I would rather collect for cancer," Will stated. "It's so much worse than diabetes."

Will and I approach our diabetes in very different ways. Will is a low-tech diabetic. When I switched to a Medtronic insulin pump over ten years ago because I was sick and tired of four insulin shots a day, Will wasn't interested. He's been injecting himself longer than I have, but he said it doesn't bother him. He's used to it.

"Shots aren't the enemy," Will explained. "I like using the Novo pens. And I couldn't stand to have something connected to me." An insulin pump delivers insulin through a thin tube under an infusion set that has to be changed every few days. "When I'm swimming or mountain-biking or making out with a girl, I don't want to think about it. It freaks me out," Will said.

You can't argue with success. Will is in great health and has excellent control of his diabetes.

When he was a high school senior, he set his mind to complete a triathlon. A rigorous training program required months of running, biking, and swimming. Will was ranked in the top group of participants. Wearing blue and yellow T-shirts emblazoned with "WILLpower," his triathlon support team lined the course on a bright, cool May morning. The race began at the high school swimming pool. We waved a huge Swedish flag, a nod to our heritage, as the swimmers took their marks and sliced down the lanes.

After the swim portion was completed, Will jumped out of the pool to get into his biking gear. We rushed to set up stations along the bike route. Our job was to provide energy drinks and protein snacks as Will looped the bicycle course at a frenzied pace. On a curve near a small lake, I watched for his bicycle and the yellow and blue T-shirt. When he came into view, I was surprised he wasn't wearing his WILLpower shirt. Instead, he was in blazing red, the American Diabetes Association's Red Rider Jersey that proudly states on the back "I RIDE WITH DIABETES!" Will, the guy who never talked about the disease, exploded out of the diabetes closet.

As he flew by me, I wept. Will didn't have to talk about diabetes. He was living it. Will finished in the top five and showed himself and everyone else that a pancreas was not required to swim, bike, run, and live life to the hilt.

During our recent conversation, I asked him why he made such a bold statement wearing the diabetes jersey on the triathlon.

"If there were kids watching the triathlon living with diabetes or other challenges, I wanted them to know they can complete a triathlon or anything else," Will replied. "It was important that I showed them through my actions rather than words."

Will has never been an outspoken diabetes advocate and we've butted heads occasionally. I've invited him to various diabetes events and he's not that interested. But a couple of summers ago, when Will was 17 he applied to be a counselor at Camp Needlepoint, the diabetes camp in Hudson, Wisconsin, where we both attended.

When he came home, he said it was a highlight for him. Here is an excerpt from Will's college essay.

"It doesn't take a cape to be a hero. I learned this when I was five years old, the year I was diagnosed with type 1 diabetes. I desperately needed a hero. I went from sliding down the snow-covered hill on a winter afternoon with my best friend, Tommy, straight to the hospital. At a very young age, my future was clouded with limitations and restrictions.

When I was ten years old, I met the fastest swimmer in the world,

Gary Hall Jr., a type 1 diabetic. He admitted that he thought his swimming career was over when he was diagnosed with diabetes. Gary even contemplated suicide. He persevered, eventually winning five Olympic gold medals—with diabetes! He inspired me to defy the odds instead of letting the disease define me.

This summer, I was a volunteer camp counselor for diabetic kids at Camp Needlepoint. The first day, I worked with a group of five-year-olds. I watched them and remembered my diagnosis, the doctors, and the hospital bed. I remember being young and scared and wondering if I would live to see my high school graduation.

My job was to show my campers how to deal with diabetes and live a normal life. I didn't just want to tell them—I wanted to give them a living example. If they needed a Gary Hall, I would be their Gary Hall.

Andy was one of my eight-year-old campers. After testing his blood, he asked me to give him a shot of insulin. Andy said his mom always did it, because he was afraid he would screw it up. I told Andy that I believed in him and knew he could do it. I walked him through the process. For the first time in the four years of having diabetes, Andy gave himself an insulin shot. It was a big deal for both of us.

Another camper, Reagan, made it clear he did not want to be at Camp Needlepoint. With his eyes red and swollen from crying, he told me being a diabetic was the hardest thing in the world. I looked him straight in the eyes. "You can do it," I said. "You have a great life ahead of you." By the end of the week, Reagan had changed dramatically. For the first time in a long time, he had a future.

Having a hero makes you want to be a hero. Gary Hall changed the way I looked at myself. He showed me how to live with a chronic illness. When things get tough, I think of Gary Hall and his refusal to surrender. I hope Andy and Reagan remember me when the going gets tough.

They're going to make great heroes."

In May 2013, Will traveled to Rwanda, Africa, for a college class on microloans. On their free day, Will persuaded the group of Baylor students to hike up the mountains with armed guards to see the famous silverback gorillas. My mom almost died when she received e-mailed photos featuring Will's wide grin in the foreground with a very large gorilla right over his shoulder. He survived that experience to return to Texas and jump out of a plane. I sometimes wonder if Will's love of life is because of diabetes or despite it. Whichever it is, it's working for him.

Over the years I've met a lot of famous and powerful people. But the one who has inspired me most is my brother Will. And it's true. It doesn't take a cape to be a hero.

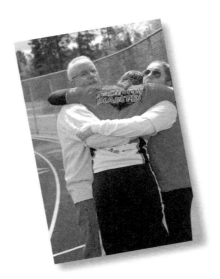

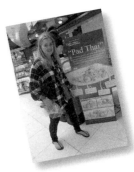

CHAPTER 16

The Diabetic Food Police

In my parent's laundry room, our school pictures march around the wall. The photos begin with kindergarten and end with senior photos. Thor's are lined up on the top. Will's are on the bottom and, as always, I'm in the middle. It's interesting to see myself age in a straight line of framed eight-by-ten-inch photos. My bottom teeth are missing in kindergarten. In first grade, they've grown in, but my top teeth are gone. Glasses in second grade. Braces from fifth to seventh grade. And a dazzling smile with straight teeth from eighth grade on.

My seventh-grade photo is in the middle of the school lineup. Wearing a purple turtleneck, my hair is pulled straight back from a pair of thick, dark eyebrows. The round face of childhood has given way to a sharp, angular face. I must have thought I looked good, because I'm flashing a confident smile, despite the hardware on my teeth. That was the last professional photograph before I was diagnosed with diabetes. I feel like taking a black marker and drawing a thick line between my seventh- and eighth-grade pictures. Before and after. I'm still smiling in eighth grade, at least for the photographer.

I remember clearly the day I was diagnosed: March 17, 1999. The doctor weighed me and noted a significant weight loss from the year before. When the pancreas no longer produces insulin, blood sugar levels are elevated and weight loss is a side effect. My blood sugar was over 700 that morning, seven times the normal level. The doctor assured me I would gain the weight back when I started to take insulin shots.

That was the last thing I needed to hear. I had an incurable disease *and* I was going to turn into a butterball. Life sucked.

I already had struggled with my weight over the previous year. I felt a certain pressure to keep it under control. As a competitive figure skater, it was a distinct advantage to weigh less. You can jump higher and spin faster with fewer pounds to move. Because I was on the tall side, I had an even more added pressure to keep my weight down. How is this going to work? Do I have to give up everything I love?

As the doctor predicted, when blood sugars fell to normal levels because of insulin shots, the lost weight returned. When diabetics experience a low blood sugar, it's treated with some type of carbohydrate to return to normal levels. There is no option. Even if you aren't hungry, you have to eat. Low blood sugars are a regular occurrence for type 1 diabetics. The worst for me come in the middle of the night. I wake up in a panic and sometimes over treat the low sugar. Instead of a single granola bar, I will have several or allow myself candy or ice cream. I'd fall back to sleep and wake up with a high blood sugar, a stomachache, and regret over the added calories.

Throughout my teenage years I continued to battle with my relationship with food. It didn't help that some misguided people assumed diabetes was a result of eating too much candy. Most people I talk to don't know the difference between the two types of diabetes, but that didn't stop a steady stream of advice.

Decades ago, diabetes experts thought it was important for diabetics to limit their sugar intake. Researchers now know that a carbohydrate is a carbohydrate whether it's a candy bar or an apple or a piece of toast. We now count carbohydrates to regulate our blood sugar. My doctor says I can eat anything in moderation. Nothing is off limits. I shouldn't be eating three of my favorite red velvet cupcakes, but neither should you.

It's hard to respond to the food police. To this day I still hear on a weekly basis, "Quinn, are you sure you should be eating that?" They are well meaning, but it just adds to the burden of the disease. And let's be honest, they are not trained medical professionals. The comments play into my insecurities. I translate the food commentary as a criticism of my weight and management of my diabetes. I am neither skinny nor fat. Rather, I'm just in the middle struggling to control a very unpredictable disease. "Are you sure you should be eating that cookie?" I've finally figured out how to answer. "I'm sorry. Is it yours?" Living with diabetes is very difficult. Don't make it any harder. The question you should be asking is, "How can I help?" That's what I would love to hear.

Body image has become a health crisis in this country. Young women and men are starving themselves to death believing thinner and thinner is better. For diabetics, it is a growing issue. I remember in junior high starving myself to be thin. What I could eat the least was the name of the game. I remember trying to stretch five saltine crackers from breakfast to dinner. Other days, maybe it was an apple. I strictly limited my insulin so I would be forced to limit my food. With diabetes, I often felt out of control. These new eating patterns were a way that I could feel in control of something. Was I the only one?

During my tenure as the youth spokesperson for the American Diabetes Association and the years after, I never heard anyone talk about eating disorders among diabetics. I attended conferences across the country, listened to top diabetes researchers and kept up on the latest trends. Not once did I hear anything about the connection between diabetes and eating disorders. Then I read a fascinating article in the *Journal of Psychosomatic Research* from 2002 titled "Eating Disorders in Young Women with Type 1 Diabetes Mellitus." The article concluded, "The prevalence rates of eating disorders amongst adolescent and young adult women with diabetes are twice as high as in their non-diabetic peers." It gave me a lot to think about. Was there a connection between my body image issues and diabetes?

In 2010, my doctor reviewed my weight chart with its wild swings over the past ten years. She suggested that I consult with a doctor who specializes in eating disorders. I was mortified. My food patterns were complicated because I had diabetes. It's hard to lose weight while managing blood sugars. I had a lot of excuses, but inside I knew I had a very unhealthy relationship with food. My life choices had brought me down a destructive path. There, in a cramped white room, the doctor told me, "Quinn, you have bulimia."

All I could do was stare back in silence. I had no words. My long blond hair, stick-straight, against my crisp, black business suit evoked an image of togetherness. With everything in me I had worked to put on a perfect front. At this moment, I just wanted to crumble up in a ball of tears on the floor and be told everything was going to be okay, but I knew it wasn't going to be that easy. I had been found out.

Melrose Center in St. Louis Park, Minnesota, collaborates with the International Diabetes Center in Park Nicollet to treat people diagnosed with an eating disorder and type 1 diabetes. After the doctor's diagnosis, I entered a treatment program and started chipping away the mask of perfectionism. I'm not a person who likes to ask for help. I pride myself on being self-sufficient. But when I hit bottom, I knew I needed help. Eating disorders paired with diabetes can be a life-threatening combination. It was a relief to be around other young women and men with diabetes who also had an eating disorder that had a stronghold on their life. I learned that there is no quick fix for diabetes or an eating disorder. Recovery is not an event; it's a daily choice.

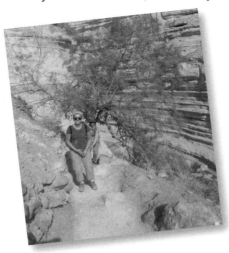

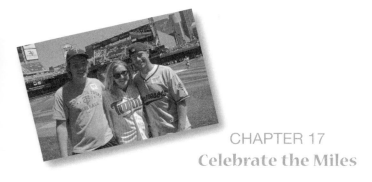

CHAPTER 17
Celebrate the Miles

People are surprised when I tell them that every year my parents celebrate the anniversary of our diabetes diagnosis. The dates are on the calendar every year, along with birthdays and wedding anniversaries. My date is March 17 and Will's is December 1. On my first-year anniversary of having diabetes, my parents asked me where I would like to go out for dinner. They gave me a big stuffed bear and a card saying how proud they were of me and how I refused to be defeated or defined by a disease. It sounds weird, but it felt really good. My Dad, a pharmacist, recognized my determination to walk through the challenge of diabetes every single day.

My mom and dad often told Will and me that they would do anything they could to help us manage our diabetes. They couldn't take the shots for us, but it made a big difference that they recognized how hard it was. When you come to my parents' house check out the family calendar and you will see D-day (diabetes day) on March 17 and December 1. There's a pair of earrings I have an eye on for my next anniversary!

Now that I'm in my twenties, friends of mine still remember my diabetes anniversary (maybe because it lands on St. Patrick's Day). They will send a card or an e-mail to encourage me. I'll never forget my tenth anniversary. I was twenty-three years old and my best friend, Kate, sent me a card telling me how she had been inspired by my journey with diabetes. At times, I've thought about what a drag it must be to have a friend who has to plan in advance when and what she needs to eat and carry around needles and insulin. Talk about a buzzkill. But Kate let me know that I was a positive example and a great friend. The diabetes journey is long and tough, but a strong family and good, supportive friends have made a huge difference in my life.

I had always wanted to go Kanakuk, a Christian sports camp in the Missouri Ozarks, and my parents agreed I could go when I turned fourteen. My cousin Shannon just two weeks younger, was going too. It was a high-energy, coed camp with every sport imaginable. We poured over the offerings, trying to decide if whitewater rafting would be more fun than rappelling or caving.

We sent our registrations in, with a request to be roommates, and got our acceptance letter. We were counting the days. Then my mother got a call from the Kanakuk nurse. Because I had type 1 diabetes, there were some safeguards and rules that I needed to sign off on. I couldn't believe I was being singled out. I read the list and stopped at the point where I was required to wear a fanny pack at all times to carry emergency food.

What would be wrong with sticking a granola bar in my pocket? Or just going to the nurse's station if I got a low blood sugar? My mom called Kanakuk to see if we could work it out, and they were adamant. The nurse said the fanny pack was necessary so staff could see that I was prepared for possible low blood sugars. She said it was a liability issue for the camp.

I cried for a week. I was devastated. Kanakuk had been a dream of mine for several years and I could not wait to go. It seemed like diabetes was the curse that just kept ruining things over and over and over. I don't want to be the designated sick girl wearing her stupid fanny pack. It wasn't worth the sick-kid label. I wouldn't go.

We were driving to Kansas City for Easter with my aunt, uncle, and cousins. I knew I would have to talk to Shannon, to let her know I wouldn't be going to Kanakuk. When we arrived at their house, Shannon and I quickly escaped to her room. We sprawled out on her double bed to catch up. Shannon talked about switching from gymnastics to the swim team and how hard the early morning practices were. Eventually the conversation turned to Kanakuk.

"I have some really bad news, Shannon."

"What's wrong?" she replied with a worried look. "What happened?"

"I can't go to Kanakuk," I whispered. "I want to, but I can't."

"Why not? You have to go. This is our year," she said. "We're registered. We are going."

I told Shannon about the nurse at Kanakuk and the list of rules including the dreaded fanny pack. "I refuse to wear a fanny pack," I said. "So they won't let me come to camp."

Shannon sympathized with me. "That is so dumb. You could carry food in your sock or your pocket. But this isn't going to stop us. We'll figure it out. Don't worry."

It was a relief to tell Shannon. She understood. I still didn't think it would ever work out, but we dropped it for the time being and went downstairs to watch a movie.

One of our favorite cousin pastimes is shopping. Shannon lived in a suburb of Kansas City with huge shopping malls, a big treat for me since I lived in the much smaller town of Brainerd, Minnesota, with Steve and Barry's anchoring the small strip mall. Mom dropped Shannon, Katelyn (Shannon's older sister), and me at the jumbo mall and said she would pick us up in four hours. It felt great to hang out with my cousins, to try on clothes, and relax.

We started at one end of the mall and worked our way around the floors. I was trying on a black-and-white polka-dot top while Katelyn was in the next dressing room with an armful of prom dresses. I came out to show Shannon my outfit and she gave it a thumbs-up. Then she turned around and modeled a sleek, black fanny pack in the small of her back.

"How cute is this?" Shannon exclaimed. "It's so cool. I'm getting it. And I think I'll wear it at Kanakuk. It's a great size for lip balm, gum and a granola bar. We will be the hippest hipsters at camp."

Holding up an identical black fanny back, Shannon exclaimed, "Thank heavens they have two of them. Kanakuk, here we come!"

I will never forget Shannon's kindness. And by the way, we had a blast at camp. Being supportive doesn't mean you have to march on Washington. Just let us know that you understand and that you care.

Nikki, an only child, was energetic and always cooking up plans for us. I loved to spend the night at her house where there were no brothers to bother us. My mom was unusually casual when I asked if I could sleep over at Nikki's.

"Sure you can go. Don't forget your sleeping bag and your insulin," she said. "I'll pick you up tomorrow. Just give me a call."

I found out later that Mom knew that Nikki's grandmother, who lived with them, was a diabetic, and the family was very familiar with the disease. As long as I could go, I didn't care.

That evening, I took the prescribed units of insulin and my blood sugar was fine until Nikki wanted to go to the Dairy Queen. I called my mom and asked if she could drive the half hour to Nikki's house with additional insulin. She refused to and suggested some low-carb snack choices that wouldn't require more insulin. I told Nikki the Dairy Queen was out for me.

Nikki came up with a great solution.

"When we play tennis, doesn't it lower your blood sugar?" she asked.

Nikki and I played doubles on the junior high tennis team. "Let's do the Tae Bo videotape and see if you can get your sugar down so we can have a Buster Bar!"

Nikki spun toward the television and gave a high kick. For the next hour, we sweated with Billy Blanks yelling at us through the TV screen. It was a blast. And the ice cream treat was delicious. Nikki came alongside me that day and helped solve a roadblock. She showed me what it meant to be a friend. Nikki didn't need to have diabetes to support me. She just needed to walk beside me.

When I talk to families of people living with diabetes, they often ask how they can be supportive. My answer is to be like my parents, or Kate, Shannon, or Nikki. Walking with us makes the journey so much easier.

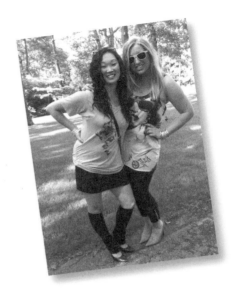

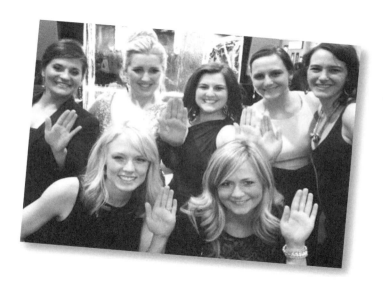

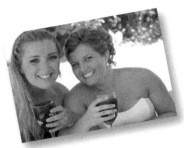

CHAPTER 18
Diabetes Dating

I will never forget when I traveled to Camp Clara Barton in Massachu-setts as the national youth advocate. After my speech, I joined people from those cabins for a bonfire barbeque. A twelve-year-old girl named Emma, freckles sprinkled across her nose, came up to me. She said she was nervous to ask her question. I told her not to worry and that she could ask me anything. With a sheepish grin, she quietly asked, "Can a girl with diabetes get a boyfriend?"

I said "Yes" instantly.

Emma replied, "Do you have a boyfriend?"

I had to confess that I didn't, but assured her I really didn't have a boyfriend before I had diabetes, so that probably wasn't the sole reason.

Emma reminded me so much of my thirteen-year-old self. The very first question I asked my doctor after I was diagnosed with diabetes wasn't about the changes I was going to have to make or how long I would live or how was I going to learn to give myself a shot. My first question was, "Can I go to the YMCA dance tonight?"

A good friend of mine, Emily, who also has type 1 diabetes, thought it was weird that I would make a big deal about telling a guy about my diabetes.

"This is a small town, Quinn, they probably already know and they don't care," she said. Emily was diagnosed at seven years old. "I can't remember when I didn't have diabetes. It's not that big of a deal to any-body but you."

Emily and Jake had been together most of high school. She said diabetes was a non-issue.

"I'm a package deal, and the guy I'm dating can take it or leave it."

It seemed so simple for Emily. I wondered why I didn't share her same sentiments. Was it because I was diagnosed in my teen years, and I remember what it was like to be Quinn without diabetes?

A friend of mine asked her steady boyfriend to wear an insulin pump (with saline, of course) for a full week so he would know what it felt like. They had talked about getting married, but Lauren wanted Matt to really understand what it was like to live with a chronic disease. You wear it twenty-four-seven, taking it off only in the shower. Matt got a glimpse of the challenges of type 1 diabetes.

Before he proposed, Lauren wanted him to know what he was signing up for. He passed the test with flying colors. They've been married for six years and doing great. Matt is what we call a "type 3 diabetic." He has a healthy pancreas but supports Lauren fully as she lives with diabetes. It's a big commitment, but he says everybody has something. Lauren can't produce insulin. It's just another challenge that they face together.

In the summer of 2013 my cousin introduced me to Andy. We were out at a bar and I ordered a Diet Coke. When the server brought it back to my table, I took a sip of it and knew that it wasn't diet. I wrinkled my nose at Katelyn. Andy grabbed the drink, walked to the bar, and asked the bartender to re-pour the drink. Andy had known me for half an hour. It was a small, but sweet, gesture. He didn't make a fuss about it, just put the newly poured Diet Coke in front of me.

In contrast, I had been set up with Connor earlier that year. We had been introduced by mutual friends, and he seemed like a great guy. On our first date, he criticized my choice of beverage: sugar-free Red Bull.

"It's terrible for you," he said. "You might get cancer down the road if you keep that up."

I was shocked. What was his problem? I explained to him that I have type 1 diabetes and that's why I choose the diet or the sugar-free option.

He quickly retorted, "That's no excuse. That stuff is so bad for you. I would never drink that."

Needless to say, we never made it to a second date. I don't need a man to chug Diet Coke with me, but I do need someone with a sensitivity chip.

Having a chronic disease is exhausting and makes life more complicated. But diabetes has made me more compassionate. I'm quick to reach out to those who struggle. At thirteen, I became independent and responsible for my life. Most important, I discovered early what my passion and purpose was in life. It took years of having diabetes to realize that the disease is just part of me—a package deal, as Emily would say. If a guy is interested in me, he has to accept the terms of my illness. If he can't get past that, he'll be the one missing out.

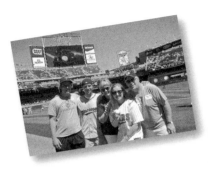

CHAPTER 19
Dear Quinn

I was running late to church on a surprisingly warm March Sunday evening in 2012. My friend Bre was saving my seat inside and I rushed inside to find her. The worship band had just finished their last song. A red-haired female pastor in her thirties announced the sermon topic: vulnerability. Without even thinking, I looked for the exit sign. I knew this was going to be too close for comfort. At twenty-seven, I had a lifetime of experience with building walls to protect myself. Some of it was probably my personality, but diabetes hadn't helped. For way too long, I'd been fighting against looking, feeling, or acting like a person with a chronic illness. I became an overachiever, desperately trying to make up for a broken body. It was exhausting, and it clearly wasn't working.

Near the end of the sermon, the pastor asked us to take out our cell phones. The church, filled with generation Xers, whipping out their phones.

"I want you to answer this question," she instructed. "If people only knew blank, they would think blank about me. Text your answer to the number on the screen."

The tension in the church crackled. You could almost hear the wheels turning. I shifted in my seat and examined my nails. Finally, I wrote down my biggest fear.

"If people only knew *how broken I am inside and what I've been through*, they would think *I'm incapable of helping others*. I hit the send button, and my eyes filled with tears. Somewhere along the road, I put on a protective coat of perfectionism. I wanted so badly to help others with their problems that I denied mine.

Looking back, I can see that speaking about my life with diabetes provided redemption. If my pain helps you, it will almost be worth it. But being a role model is a heavy load to carry. Somewhere along the way, I lost my way. I lost myself.

Living with a chronic illness became the center of my world and every decision was built on that reality. My pancreas, an ugly little organ the size of my fist, stopped working one day. Science cannot explain why it happened to me. I didn't cause it. So why do I keep blaming myself? Sitting in the darkened church, I realized that everyone around me had something that they had to overcome in their life. Every single one of us is less than what we aspire to be. We are all broken.

God has used everything in my life—from the mountaintops to the valleys—to shape me into the person I am today. My life is so much more than diabetes. I am a devoted friend, daughter, and sister. I am passionate about God, traveling, figure skating, popcorn, and polka dots. Diabetes is not a headline in my life. It's a footnote.

I'd like to close this journal by writing a letter to my thirteen-year-old self who desperately needed hope and strength on March 17, 1999.

Dear Quinn,

Life is unpredictable. You can't control this sharp turn that life has taken. Telling you that diabetes is no big deal won't help. It is a big deal. Diabetes is a chronic, incurable illness that you will have to consider every day for the rest of your life. The good news is you still have choices. Trust me. Your parents may want to keep you safe and sound, bubble-wrapped with perfect blood sugar levels. Resist. Don't let anyone limit your future. Diabetes cannot destroy your dreams unless you let it.

Taking off the outer protection will make you a target at times. You are different. You carry a burden. But don't ever forget that others carry burdens too. Be gentle with them. Be gentle with yourself.

Fear can be crippling, debilitating at times. How is this going to turn out? Will I be able to….(fill in the blank)? The shame you might feel after being diagnosed can be overwhelming, overshadowing your present and future. Pray. Breathe through it. It too shall pass. Diabetes will teach you that you cannot do life on your own; you will simply not make it. Most people realize this at some point in their lives. For us, we just found out sooner.

Remember your heroes. You can't be a hero if you don't have challenges to overcome. Your Grandpa Gordon was a great adventurer and well known for his ocean-sailing adventures. When his wife or adult children protested that it was too risky, he explained his philosophy of life.

"I could get up every morning and go down to the basement to lie between two mattresses," Grandpa said. "At the end of the day, I would be safe and sound, but what kind of quality of life is that?" He refused to live like that. Grandpa died last year but he lived, eighty-five years old and well-satisfied.

That's how you live your life with diabetes. Manage what you can, but don't refuse to participate in life because your pancreas quit. You may not be able to see it now, but you have a big life ahead of you. Ride elephants in Thailand. Dance with the Maasai in Tanzania. Blow through a triathlon. Float in the Dead Sea. Even write a book. Diabetes cannot kill your dreams. Only you can do that. CAN is a powerful word.

You may get beaten and bruised along your journey. Friends and family let you down. Crushing challenges are forced on you before you are mature enough or strong enough to handle them. You shed tears and wonder why life has to be so hard. You think that you can't survive diabetes. But you are wrong. You are stronger and more determined than you know. Look around. We are all terminal. Living with an incurable disease helps us focus on quality rather than quantity.

Surround yourself with family and friends who speak truth and love into your life. When you can't take another step, they will come alongside you to help you. Fix your eyes on God and pray for the strength to walk the path before you. And keep walking.

Love Always,
Quinn

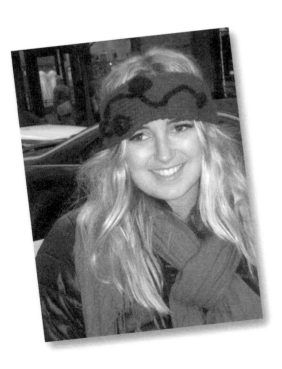

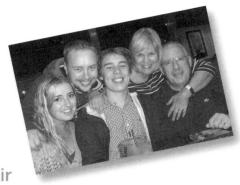

A Note from Quinn's Mother
Diabetes...A Family Affair
by Rachel Reabe Nystrom

It just up and quit. No reason, no warning, no explanation. Will's pancreas stopped producing insulin. One day our five-year-old son was sliding down the snowy hill behind our house and the next he was in the hospital learning how to live the rest of his life with diabetes, an incurable disease.

Life as we knew it was over. The first time I had to put a hypodermic needle into Will's sweet, soft arm, I sobbed my heart out. I cried for Will and for our family and a future that seemed beyond bleak. And then we kept going, because the only options were life or death.

An upcoming family vacation became a survival test. Could we manage diabetes away from our home and doctor? The tiny bottle of insulin was guarded more carefully than our wallet or passports. We could live without the latter but Will could not survive without insulin. Bob and I each wore a small pouch around our necks with insulin vials. Our time was an unqualified success. Life was not the same but it could be managed and enjoyed. We stopped holding our breath and tried to allow Will to be a five-year-old boy.

Three years later our thirteen-year-old daughter, Quinn, was diagnosed with diabetes. With no family history of diabetes, it seemed impossible. The good news was, we knew how to live with diabetes. The bad news was, we knew how to live with diabetes. I cried out to God, convinced that I had flunked His first test, requiring a retake at Quinn's expense. He came close in those dark days, reassuring us of His love and faithfulness.

Life rolled along in a new normal way. Insulin shots and blood sugar checks four times a day were wedged in between school and church and friends and hockey and figure skating and sleepovers. Will and Quinn got used to managing their insulin doses. Thor, our oldest child, was the odd man out. The only kid who didn't have to take an insulin shot before meals.

Finding a cure for diabetes became a very personal issue. We got involved with the American Diabetes Association and put together a team for the annual Walk for Diabetes. We were overwhelmed by the generosity of our families and friends. When Will was diagnosed with diabetes, Quinn pledged to work the rest of her life to help find a cure. Later, as a bona fide diabetic, she redoubled her efforts, pulling the rest of us along in her considerable wake.

Will and Quinn joined other young diabetics across the country in Washington, DC to lobby Congress for increased funding for diabetes. They shared their stories of living with diabetes with United States senators and representatives. It was exhilarating for a couple of kids from Minnesota. They began to believe they could make a difference.

Along the way, Quinn and Will found heroes. Will met Gold Olympian Gary the fastest swimmer on earth and a diabetic. Quinn forged a friendship with Nicole Johnson, the only Miss America in history with a chronic disease, diabetes.

Our kids also became heroes. Quinn developed relationships with younger girls in our community with diabetes, cheering them on and challenging them to make the most of their lives. Will was a counselor at a diabetes camp last summer. He helped young boys understand that diabetes only limits life if they let it. He urged them to take control of their disease by managing their insulin shots and blood sugars. But mostly, he showed them how to have crazy fun despite diabetes.

Quinn and Will went off to college packing laptops, bikes and a generous supply of needles, insulin and blood testing supplies. "Don't worry, Mom." I forced a confident smile and assured them I was not worried. Meanwhile, I calculated how fast I could get to Holland, Michigan or Waco, Texas in an emergency. I'm happy to report, we all survived.

Despite their chronic illness or perhaps because of it, both Quinn and Will are adventurers. Quinn studied in Tanzania and explored the jungles of Thailand on an elephant. This year Will climbed the Great Wall of China, survived a close encounter with a silverback gorilla in Rwanda and tried skydiving. Sometimes diabetes is the least of my worries.

Diabetes has brought us close as a family. Our faith is deeper and our understanding of God clearer. Our children learned compassion. They know how it feels to struggle and they're willing to reach out to others. They don't give up easily. The harder road isn't impossible, it is just harder. Quinn and Will understand that diabetes does not have the power to determine their quality of life. That's a choice they get to make.